D0934856

A Doctor's Guide to Feeding Your Child

A Doctor's Guide

COMPLETE NUTRITION

Stephen J. Atwood, M.D.

to Feeding Your Child

FOR HEALTHY GROWTH

MACMILLAN PUBLISHING CO., INC.
NEW YORK

COLLIER MACMILLAN PUBLISHERS
LONDON

Copyright © 1982 by Stephen J. Atwood, M.D.

All rights reserved. No part of this book may be reproduced or transmitted in any form or by any means, electronic or mechanical, including photocopying, recording or by any information storage and retrieval system, without permission in writing from the Publisher.

Macmillan Publishing Co., Inc.
866 Third Avenue, New York, N.Y. 10022
Collier Macmillan Canada, Inc.

Library of Congress Cataloging in Publication Data

Atwood, Stephen J.
   A doctor's guide to feeding your child.

   Includes index.
      1. Children—Nutrition.   2. Nutrition disorders
in children.   I. Title.
RJ206.A88   649'.3   82-15248
ISBN 0-02-504400-1   AACR2

10   9   8   7   6   5   4   3   2

Printed in the United States of America

To my father, my sister, and
especially to Carmen,
for their teaching, patience,
and love

Contents

Preface

IN MY YEARS AS A MEDICAL EDUCATOR, I have had the opportunity to teach nutrition to hundreds of students, interns, residents, and practitioners. I teach pediatrics, which is almost the same thing as saying that I teach child nutrition. I am also a practicing pediatrician, interested in children's growth and development; and nutrition and growth and development are, as you will read, so integrally related that a discussion of one requires discussion of the other.

Child nutrition has, over the years, become of increasing concern and interest to the medical profession. Our journals regularly contain informative articles on the subject and give us reports of studies and research in the field. We talk about developments in child nutrition in our medical conferences and as we make our rounds in teaching hospitals. But when, as a practicing pediatrician, I talk with parents and patients, I all too often find that this information is not reaching them. Or, if it is reaching them, it is being misinterpreted. My primary motivation for writing this book was to bring the information to those for whose welfare it is intended, and to do so as clearly and understandably as possible.

When I sit with a mother in my office explaining, say, why her baby does not need supplemental iron until the age of four or five months, I realize that I am not the primary physician here. The mother is. She is the one who is ultimately responsible for her child's nutritional welfare. Similarly, when I advise an adolescent about the dangers of a fad or crash diet, I know that the ultimate responsibility for his or her dietary regimen is not mine. It is the patient's. My responsibility is to see to it that parents and patients *understand the reasons for* my advice. If they do not, they are unlikely to take it as seriously as I would hope.

And why should they? The days of doing something just because the doctor says so have passed. Many of my medical forebears believed that explanations merely confused the patient, that, in any case, the patient couldn't understand them. I have not found this to be true. The parents and teenagers I talk to today want to know the rationale behind the medical advice I give them. They want to know why. And they are perfectly capable of understanding the principles of good nutrition.

So in this book I have tried to supply reasons for the advice I give. I do not talk down to the parents or patients. I assume that the reader wants to know the *why* as well as the *how* of good nutrition.

The book is divided into two parts. Part One presents an overview of the basics of nutritional science. It covers normal child nutrition, in relation to biochemical and physiological development of the child, from the prenatal period through adolescence. Part Two focusses on specific nutritional problems. Some of these problems are very serious. Others, less so. All of them, however, when and if they arise, should be dealt with promptly.

Much of the book is written in dialogue form, partly because I feel this stylistic device gives more immediacy to the information I wish to convey, and partly because I feel more at home with it—the clinical questions about normal and abnormal nutrition arose from my conversations with parents. My training as a pediatrician has supplied me with the body of knowledge necessary for answering those questions. My care and concern for the total health of my patients and my sense of responsibility to their parents have been my motive for teaching.

Acknowledgments

I would like to offer special gratitude to Dr. Fred Agre for his advice; Maudene Nelson for the preparation of the various menus; Gisele Thornhill and also Amy Laskin and Robert Stewart for their help in preparing the manuscript at various stages in its development; Jeanine and Bill Reilly and the other parents and patients who have taught me so much; and particularly Jane Cullen and Toni Lopopolo for their persistent patience and direction.

PART I
Your Child's Normal Nutrition

CHAPTER 1

Prenatal Concerns

WHEN I FIRST MET Mrs. Richardson she was in the thirtieth week of her pregnancy. She questioned me about her weight gain during her pregnancy. The questions, however, were really about feeding her unborn baby. After all, what nourished her, nourished the baby. In fact, at its own expense if necessary, her body would automatically preserve her baby's growth and protect its well-being.

The growth of a baby in the womb is accomplished with such deceptive ease that one is unlikely to hear expectant mothers and fathers talking about what to feed the fetus tonight, when to start sending iron through the placenta, is it getting its calcium, and so forth. As long as the mother eats well and stays healthy, production continues on schedule. Yet, prenatal nutrition is an important concern. The relentless growth of the fetus puts a significant nutritional burden on the mother. She grows to a size that feels too large; she notices changes in her body and metabolism that seem out of her control.

The expectant mother wants to know if she is eating the right or the wrong food. Her concern is understandable. She may even be more anxious before birth than after, since she cannot take a look inside her body to make sure everything is going well.

Questions about feeding her baby after it is born—about breast-feeding versus bottle-feeding, for example—are usually asked as the pregnancy nears its completion. As the baby's pediatrician, I like to get involved at this point. Fundamental decisions about the first months of life can and should be made before the birth. I try to meet with the parents in this quiet period, usually one or two months before the expected arrival.

"Dr. Atwood, my name is Lucille Richardson. I have a friend down the street who told me to call you. I wonder if my husband and I could sit down with you in the next few weeks and talk to you about the birth of our child, which could happen— I guess in a couple of months!" She laughed happily. We arranged to meet in two weeks.

Mrs. Richardson came alone to see me the first time. Her husband had been unexpectedly called out of town. When I saw her she certainly looked all of thirty weeks pregnant. Everything was going according to schedule with no complications. Her blood pressure was normal; she said she had been neither smoking nor drinking during the pregnancy. She was happily excited and felt great.

Weight Gain During Pregnancy

Although her weight gain had been appropriate, her first concern was that she had gained too much. "I feel so fat!" she complained. "I've already gained 17 pounds, and my obstetrician tells me I've got two months more to go. I'm sure she's wrong. Everyone says I look as though I'm going to deliver tomorrow."

"What does she say about your weight gain so far?" I asked.

"She says it's fine. That it's not so much the amount of weight I put on—within reason, of course—but when I put it on that's most important. She says I should count on gaining anywhere from 20 to 25 pounds during the pregnancy."

"And that seems like a lot to you," I said.

"Yes, that seems like too much. You know, I saw a friend of mine the other day who hasn't lost any of the weight she put on during her pregnancy. And her baby's already four months old."

"That happens to some women. But you have to ask a few questions. What did she weigh before, and how much weight did she gain during the pregnancy?"

"Well, she was a little overweight," Mrs. Richardson admitted, "and she told me she had gained close to 35 pounds."

"Did she breast-feed her baby?" I asked.

"No. But I'm not sure I understand how this applies to her being too fat."

"Let me explain," I said. "First of all . . ."

Mrs. Richardson's concerns are certainly familiar ones and her questions valid. Most new mothers are anxious about the distortion in body image that being pregnant can generate. Many find this distortion rather easy to deal with, particularly since the reward at the end of pregnancy is such a great one. But even some of these mothers sometimes wonder if they'll ever be the same as far as their physical condition in general and their attractiveness in particular are concerned. It is hardly comforting when so many pounds are gained so easily during pregnancy. Why 25 pounds? Even if the baby weighs 9 pounds, that leaves an excess of 16 pounds to deal with after the pregnancy. Where does it go? Wouldn't it be better to gain only the bare minimum—maybe 10 to 15 pounds?

The answers to such questions have come from recent research into fetal growth by doctors and nutritionists who studied the problem of small babies, infant deaths, and a condition called "intrauterine growth retardation"—sometimes abbreviated IUGR. Intrauterine growth retardation means poor growth of the fetus while it's in the womb. Concern about the size of the fetus comes from evidence that very small babies (under 4½ pounds) are more likely to do poorly after birth. Intrauterine growth retardation results in very small babies who are at greater risk of dying in the first month of life or of developing poorly later.

There are many causes of IUGR—smoking during pregnancy, excessive alcohol or other drug consumption, and malnutrition are some examples. All such causes have to do with the balance between the demands of the fetus and the supplies provided by the mother. The center of this supply-and-demand balance is the placenta. Insufficient supplies from the mother (as when she is severely undernourished) are reflected in a small placenta. A small placenta leads to a small fetus. The excessive growth of a baby of a diabetic mother is equally dangerous. In this case the fetus "outgrows the placenta," particularly if it stays in the womb too long.

By studying the causes of these abnormalities in growth and development, doctors have come to know what is necessary for normal growth and development. As I explained to Mrs. Richardson, her obstetrician was right, and certainly up to date on the latest medical literature. She needs to gain 25 pounds (equivalent to 12 kilograms) during her pregnancy to insure the adequate nutrition and growth of her baby. Not all of the weight gained goes directly to the fetus, and this is where the confusion arises. Early in pregnancy, weight gain provides the mother with energy stores for the pregnancy and for lactation afterward. It goes toward growth of the uterus and growth of the breasts. Weight gained later in the pregnancy is for the fetus and the placenta. Since the sequence is predetermined, the timing of weight gain is important.

"From what we've learned," I told Mrs. Richardson, "you're doing you and your baby a favor by putting on most of the 25 pounds in the last six months of your pregnancy, the second and third trimesters. A mother should plan to gain just under 4 pounds a month during that period—that's almost a pound a week. Remember, the weight gained in the second trimester goes toward preparing your body for the pregnancy and for breast-feeding after pregnancy. It is roughly distributed as 1 to 2 pounds for your uterus, 1 to 2 pounds for your breasts, 1 to 2 pounds for an increase in your blood volume, plus a deposit of roughly 10 pounds of energy in the form of fats."

"Ten pounds of fat?!" she exclaimed. "But that's exactly what a mother doesn't want. It took me long enough to lose 5 pounds when I wanted to. How will I ever get rid of 10?"

"I understand," I said. "But believe me, almost all of that fat will go toward—in fact, is *necessary* for—the energy needed for lactation. You'll burn it off in the first two or three months if you breast-feed your baby. That's one of the reasons your friend had trouble losing all that weight she gained," I continued. "She didn't breast-feed. A newborn baby eats close to 500 calories a day, and those calories come from those fat stores. And your body uses up other calories in preparing those calories for the baby. When you breast-feed you use a lot of energy, and the body finds it very important to store up those calories of energy in advance—so important that it will go ahead with it even if it means there won't be enough for normal fetal growth in the last trimester."

"Do I have to worry about that?" she asked.

I explained that she didn't, as long as she added the necessary weight during the pregnancy. Mrs. Richardson was not malnourished to begin with. If she had been underweight, she would have had to gain more than 25 pounds. If she had been overweight, her requirements for weight gain during pregnancy would be slightly reduced, but no less than 15 pounds.

"The weight gained in the last trimester goes specifically toward the baby," I continued. "Seven to 8 pounds to the fetus, 1 to 2 pounds to the placenta. The amniotic fluid weighs about 1 pound. That's why it isn't good to try to lose weight in those last few months. The growing baby needs that food for life in the womb."

"But you *can* get too fat, can't you?" she asked.

"Yes, you can, and you may run into problems with high

blood pressure if you do. This condition is called eclampsia. And some mothers may develop diabetes. The warning signal here is if you're gaining more than 6 or 7 pounds a month in the last two trimesters. I don't think you have to worry about that. By my calculation, you're right on schedule."

"Should I have been on a special diet through all of this?" she asked. "I mean, some things you read make you feel as if you should open a drugstore in order to eat right for your baby—vitamin pills, calcium pills, magnesium. What should you take?"

"There are a few guidelines you can use," I said.

Nutritional Requirements During Pregnancy

Basically, the nutritional requirements for pregnancy can be met by increasing the intake of a normal *balanced* diet by 300 to 500 calories a day. Thus, if Mrs. Richardson simply takes her normal, well-balanced diet and increases it by 300 to 500 calories each day, she will receive all of the nutrients she needs for her own health and for her baby's growth.

The key words in this statement are "balanced diet." If her regular diet does not contain enough protein (not enough meats, fish, poultry, certain grains), the fetus will grow at the mother's expense, using her protein for its growth. This would also happen if all her additional calories were in the form of carbohydrates. A *balanced* increase in her diet will provide the additional protein which she requires.

She must also be sure that her diet has enough iron, calcium and folic acid in it. Iron is a mineral essential for blood formation and for the action of certain enzymes and is therefore important for her own increased blood production and for the fetus. As in the case of protein, however, the fetus' requirements come first. If the mother does not take in enough iron, *she*—not the fetus—will become iron deficient. Calcium is necessary for the development of the bones in the fetal skeleton. Mrs. Richardson will not have to worry about taking calcium pills, however, since the absorption of the calcium already in her diet, particularly in milk and cheese, will be increased. Our bodies absorb more calcium when more calcium is needed. Nutritionists point out, however, that if we consume too much phosphorus, which can be found excessively in some carbonated soft drinks, we don't absorb calcium as well. Folic acid goes into the production of new cells. It is found abundantly in the normal diet. It is also produced in sufficient quantity for a nonpregnant person by the action of bacteria on food in our intestines. The demands of a growing fetus, however, may overwhelm this natural supply, requiring that the mother increase her intake of folic acid.

"I know that you get iron in meats, fish, and egg yolks and from some vegetables," Mrs. Richardson said, "and I know that there's a lot of calcium in milk. But where do you get folic acid? What foods should I eat if I want to get more of it that way?"

"You'll find a lot of folic acid in liver, in yeast, and in dark green leafy vegetables," I said. "Liver is also a good source of iron."

"Let me get something clear, then," she went on. "Are you saying that if I had simply increased my diet 300 to 500 calories a day by drinking milk and eating the usual meats, vegetables, bread, fruit, and other sources of carbohydrates, I wouldn't have had to take any vitamins or iron pills?"

"Technically, that's right," I said, "although I still recommend the iron pills since it's difficult to tell when we're really iron deficient. Anemia may be a late sign, coming after other aspects of metabolism have been affected."

"How much iron?" she asked.

"I recommend 300 mg of ferrous sulfate once or twice a day. The reason this is all you need is that you were well nourished to begin with."

There are only a few circumstances I can think of under which I would recommend adding vitamins and calcium to a woman's diet: a mother from an impoverished family whose nutrition has been chronically poor, a pregnant teenager who has just completed her own growth spurt, an expectant mother who has been ill, with accompanying poor nutrition. Mrs. Richardson did not fit any of these descriptions. My reluctance to recommend vitamin pills to mothers who do not need them arises from my experience with some mothers who took them and then felt less compelled to eat well, assuming, incorrectly, that the pills would answer all their needs.

"What about magnesium?" she asked. "Isn't magnesium as necessary for growth as calcium and phosphorus?"

"Actually, it's important for energy production. It's used in something called oxidative phosphorylation—an important biochemical pathway that allows for storage of energy in the body and is, therefore, very important for growth."

"How do I know I'm getting enough of it?" she asked.

"Well, that's just it. It's like vitamin A, vitamin D, vitamin C and the others. If you're eating a well-balanced diet you'll get enough of all of them."

"And if you don't eat enough, is it really bad for the baby?" she asked.

As I explained to Mrs. Richardson, it does seem to be true that if a mother is severely malnourished during her pregnancy, her child will be smaller than normal at birth. And it is true that a small-for-gestational-age baby, as the very small baby is sometimes called, may have more growth and developmental problems later in life. However, the growth and normal development of the child depend on events occurring during the pregnancy *and* in the first years after birth. Inadequacies of nutrition during pregnancy may sometimes be compensated for in the first year or even two years of life. Adequate nutrition during this time results in the so-called catch-up growth seen in premature infants and some small-for-gestational-age infants. This catching up gives the baby a wider margin of safety in terms of growth, and it also underscores the importance of postnatal nutrition. The child whose chances for normal growth and development are best is the one who is adequately nourished before and after birth.

"Which brings up another point," Mrs. Richardson began. "I think I'd like to breast-feed, but I've got a lot of questions about it. I want to keep working after the baby is born. Will I be able to and still breast-feed? I hear it ruins your figure, too."

"It's best if I talk with you *and* your husband about this," I replied. "Can we make an appointment for another time and talk about it then? Make sure your husband can come, too."

CHAPTER 2

Selecting Your Baby's Nutrition

Bottle-Feeding or Breast-Feeding: Making the Decision

Mrs. Richardson returned in two weeks with her husband, who was obviously pleased that I wanted to talk to him. He had his own questions about their baby-to-be, and especially about breast-feeding and bottle-feeding.

The decision to breast-feed or bottle-feed is an important one and should ideally be made only with the knowledge and consent of both parents. Success of their choice will depend on their cooperation and mutual support. If the parents are divided on the question, success is unlikely and the guilt that accompanies failure is virtually guaranteed.

Except in unusual circumstances, I strongly advise parents to breast-feed their baby for the first four to six months. Should it be impossible to sustain breast-feeding for that long a period, I suggest they do it as long as they can. My experience has convinced me that any breast-feeding is better for the baby than no breast-feeding.

All of this is fine, but I am not the parent. There is no reason

why parents like the Richardsons should take my advice unless I assume the responsibility for making sure they understand what breast-feeding is all about—why I believe it is good
for their baby and for them, why it is superior to bottle-feeding and, also, the problems that may be involved.

"Why is breast-feeding better than bottle-feeding for our
baby?" was Mrs. Richardson's first question. She was asking
a question that would never have been raised a century ago,
before the advent of infant formulas as we know them. She
was also expressing a willingness to consider the choice between two reasonable, although not equal, alternatives for infant feeding.

There are actually a number of reasons why breast-feeding
and breast milk are better than bottle-feeding and formulas.
Some of them have been newly discovered, like the enhanced
protection against respiratory and intestinal infections con-
ferred by breast milk. Some of them have been known or observed for hundreds of years, like the easier digestibility of
breast milk and the presence of less curd in the spitting up of
breast-fed babies. And some of them have been known intu-
itively for centuries, but only recently explained by scientific
inquiry—the fact, for example, that breast milk from a well-
nourished mother has all of the nutrients necessary for normal
growth and can be the sole element in the baby's diet for as
long as six months.

I began my discussion about breast-feeding with the Richardsons with one item of age-old knowledge: the easier digestibility of breast milk.

Nutritional Differences Between
Breast Milk, Cow's Milk, and Formula

"Now remember," I said, "most of the arguments in the past
compared breast milk to cow's milk. Cow's milk never wins in
that argument. Our ancestors knew that, which is why they
turned to goat's milk or ass's milk rather than cow's milk

whenever they could. Both are more like human milk in their protein composition, and hence more digestible. Modern day pharmaceutical companies which manufacture infant formulas have made their formulas less like cow's milk and as much like human milk as possible. That should tell you something to begin with.

"In order to understand what formulas are all about," I explained to the Richardsons, "you should know the differences between mature human milk and cow's milk. And then we'll talk about where the infant formulas fit in." I showed them a chart which I keep handy for such occasions and asked them to look it over:

	% Protein	% Fat	% Carbo.	Na (mEq./L)	Ca/P	Renal Solute Load
Cow's Milk	20	51	29	25	1.3/1	220
Human Milk	7	51	42	7	2.1/1	81
Formula	9	50	41	12	1.2/1	110

I went on to explain that in the nineteenth century, formulas were made with cow's milk and water after it had been recognized that cow's milk had too much protein in the form of casein. When cow's milk was left to stand or treated with acid, it would separate into a cheesy coagulum—the curd—and a thin liquid—the whey. Casein protein is contained in the curd. Whey contains different types of milk protein, easier for babies to digest. Little Miss Muffet could sit on her tuffet and eat her curds and whey (a sort of junket or dessert) without ill effect, because she was old enough to digest both types of protein, casein and whey. But with so much more casein than whey in cow's milk, a baby cannot do so. Breast milk, with its lesser quantity of casein, forms hardly any curd when treated with acid in a test tube—or in the baby's stomach, where the "experiment" was originally performed. When the baby spit up breast milk, there was no curd; when the baby spit up cow's milk, the difference was obvious.

"Couldn't some of the protein have been removed from the cow's milk?" Mrs. Richardson asked.

"Technology was not advanced enough to allow that," I said. "So the early pediatricians tried the next best thing: they diluted the milk with water to reduce the casein concentration. Of course, by doing so they also diluted the calories, fats and carbohydrates and they diluted the whey proteins by the same amount. They did add cane sugar for calories and carbohydrates, and occasionally cream for fat, to their watered-down solution. But it has only been with modern technology that scientists have been able to add whey without casein, so that now a large part of the protein in formulas is whey protein."

"Is this just a long way of telling us that the protein in modern formulas is fine and just like that in breast milk?" asked Mrs. Richardson.

"I left out one thing: that the proteins in breast milk and cow's milk are different in quantity *and* in quality. The type of proteins in cow's milk whey is different from that in breast milk whey, so that even after the modification in amount of protein and proportion of casein to whey, cow's milk is still more appropriate for the needs of growing cows, and breast milk for the needs of growing infants."

"I notice on the chart," said Mr. Richardson, "that the amount of fat in cow's milk, human milk, and formula is roughly the same. Is this like protein: even where the quantity is the same, the products differ?"

"Yes, and the question is an important one," I answered. "Cow's milk butterfat is not as well absorbed as the fats found in human milk and in vegetable oils. If you feed an infant too much butterfat, a large part of it will be passed unabsorbed through the intestines. The baby's stools will be large, greasy, and foul smelling, which means that the infant is losing a lot of calories by that route alone. Babies fed human milk fat absorb 85 to 90 percent of it, so you can see that not much is wasted in the stools.

"Vegetable oils," I went on, "are absorbed almost as completely as human milk fats, which is why they are being used in modern formulas. Vegetable oils have a lot of what are called polyunsaturated fatty acids; more than breast milk. Vegetable oils are also very low in cholesterol."

"Isn't that supposed to be good?" asked Mr. Richardson. "Aren't we all supposed to be eating less saturated fatty acids and less cholesterol to prevent heart disease?"

Mr. Richardson's confusion goes to the heart of a major controversy. Although a high polyunsaturated fatty acid and low cholesterol diet may be good for adults, no one is entirely sure about the effect of such a diet on a growing baby. Some explanation must be made for the relatively high concentration of cholesterol in both early and mature breast milk. How has it survived the evolutionary process if it is not in some way beneficial for survival?

Humans are capable of manufacturing their own cholesterol. It might be that in babies this cholesterol should be supplemented by more cholesterol in the diet since babies are rapidly producing new nerve cells and new bile salts, both of which require cholesterol for their synthesis. Some researchers hypothesize that internal manufacture of cholesterol might only marginally meet the demand and that this is the reason breast milk has a relatively high concentration. Another, as yet unproven, explanation is that cholesterol in the diet early in life stimulates enzymes which will be important for the metabolism of cholesterol later in life. Experimental results testing these hypotheses are as yet contradictory and inconclusive.

The different types of fat in cow's milk and formulas have other effects as well. It is known that a child on a diet high in polyunsaturated fatty acids, such as those found in formulas, should have the diet supplemented with foods rich in vitamin E (widely distributed in green plants, particularly wheat cereals and added to formulas), since vitamin E is not easily absorbed in the presence of polyunsaturated fats. It has also been pointed out that vegetable oils from corn and soy have two to three times more essential fatty acids than does breast milk. Essential fatty acids are important for metabolism and are called "essential" because they cannot be made by the body and so *must* be contained in the diet. (Cow's milk fat contains only a quarter of the essential fatty acid found in breast milk.) The as yet unanswered question is: what is the effect of such a *large* amount of essential fatty acids on the growing infant?

"Do you think it's dangerous?" asked Mr. Richardson.

"I don't know," I answered. "But when one slice of the pie is cut too large, another slice has to be made smaller if you are to have the same number of slices. A baby can only eat so much. Too much linoleic acid (that's the essential fatty acid we're talking about) means less of something else."

"So," said Mrs. Richardson, "once again it appears that breast milk is somewhat better than formula and certainly better than cow's milk in the fats and cholesterol category."

"I'd say so."

"And carbohydrates?" she asked.

I explained that the carbohydrate in both cow's milk and in breast milk is lactose, and that the only difference between the two is the amount, a difference taken into account by the pharmaceutical companies in their preparation of infant formulas. In some vegetable-protein formulas which are intended for the occasional child who has cow's milk protein allergy, a different type of sugar, such as dextrose or sucrose, is used, since the lactose occasionally contains some trace of the cow's milk protein.

"The ratio of calcium to phosphorus," Mr. Richardson pointed out, "is certainly different in cow's milk and breast milk. And there seems to have been no attempt to change it in the infant formula. Is that as significant as the ratio of casein to whey?"

"No. In fact the significance of the calcium/phosphorus ratio is very cloudy. It used to be thought that a calcium/phosphorus ratio of 2 to 1, as found in breast milk, was ideal and made the absorption of calcium from the intestines more efficient. But this was based on animal experiments and never proven conclusively in humans. We probably enjoy a wider range of safety when it comes to calcium and phosphorus absorption. The 1980 *Recommended Dietary Allowances,* prepared by the National Research Council, recommends a calcium/phosphorus ratio in the range of 1 to 1 or slightly greater."

"I remember your telling me about too much phosphorus from some soft drinks interfering with calcium absorption," said Mrs. Richardson. "Doesn't that apply here?"

"It does, but only if the amount of phosphorus is significantly greater than the calcium, which would cause the calcium/phosphorus ratio to be considerably less than one. If there were twice as much phosphorus, for instance, Ca/P would be $\frac{1}{2}$, or .5. That could result either from drinking a lot of soft drinks or from not eating enough calcium, or from both. One other thing I should mention is that the total amount of calcium in human milk, although considerably less than in cow's milk, is sufficient for growth because it is so well absorbed. Increased amounts of lactose apparently enhance calcium absorption, and human milk contains slightly more lactose than cow's milk. An infant fed human milk absorbs 65 to 70 percent of the calcium provided. On the other hand, an infant will absorb only 25 to 30 percent of the amount of calcium in cow's milk."

"Hm," said Mr. Richardson, scanning the chart like a businessman reviewing his investments. "Cow's milk sodium 25, Human milk sodium 7." He looked up at me. "Less salt in human milk?"

I nodded.

"And what's this column 'renal solute load'?" he asked, pointing to the last column on the chart.

In order to answer Mr. Richardson's question, a review of some basic concepts was in order. The internal environment of the body, I explained, is carefully maintained in a state of equilibrium called *homeostasis,* which translates roughly from the Greek to mean "standing the same." This equilibrium is extremely important. For example, our heartbeat becomes irregular and may even stop if our potassium level becomes too high or too low. If we retain too much sodium in our blood, we may develop high blood pressure; if blood sodium drops suddenly, our brain cells will swell. If our serum urea (urea is a compound occurring in body fluids as a product of protein metabolism) rises above normal levels, we become confused and may even go into a coma. The equilibrium represents a balance between what we take in and what we put out.

The organ probably most important for maintaining this balance is our kidney. (Functions which the kidney performs are called renal functions.) If we take in too much potassium, our kidneys filter the excess out of the blood and excrete it in the urine. If we consume too little, the filter is functionally closed down and we retain potassium. The same is true for sodium, chloride, and urea. (Some calcium homeostasis is regulated by the kidneys, but most is controlled by the absorption of dietary calcium from the bowel: when we need more, more is absorbed and when we need less, less is absorbed. Calcium in the blood is also in balance with calcium in the bones. If the serum calcium begins to drop, more calcium is released from its storage in the bones.)

In order for these solutes, as the sodium, potassium, chloride, and urea are called, to be excreted in the urine they must be diluted in a certain amount of water—water, after all, is what makes up the large part of urine. In adults and children beyond infancy, the amount of water excreted also depends on the needs for internal balance. If we are becoming dehydrated because of vomiting, diarrhea, sweating, or simply not drinking enough, our kidneys respond by saving water; less is excreted and our urine becomes more concentrated—truly a lifesaving mechanism. There is a problem, however, with the newborn and young infant. Their kidneys have not yet developed the ability to respond to dehydration by saving water and concentrating the urine. In some children the kidney will not be mature enough to do this until almost a year of age.

This means that the infant who has a high solute load which must be excreted in order to maintain homeostasis must do so with an obligatory and relatively uncontrollable loss of water. In this case, the only thing that regulates the amount of water lost is the amount of solute delivered to the kidneys. If the solute load is high, a lot of water gets excreted, even if the child is becoming dehydrated from an ongoing diarrhea or from not getting enough fluids.

"This obviously would have a bad effect on the child," said Mrs. Richardson. "What about your theory that normal body functions have evolved because they have a beneficial effect on survival?"

"Well, it means that a diet high in these solutes is *not* conducive to normal body function," I answered. "Which is why foods that lead to a high renal solute load . . ."

"Like cow's milk," interrupted Mr. Richardson, referring to the chart.

"Like cow's milk," I agreed, "and like solid foods. Both should be avoided in early infancy. But we'll talk more about that later. Formula companies have recognized the importance of renal solute load and have reduced it in their formulas to a more manageable amount. They've also lowered the sodium content in their formulas because of its contribution to renal solute load and its possible effect on the later development of high blood pressure. But this is another nutritional area in which research has yet to provide a clear answer."

"The differences between cow's milk and human milk are enormous, as you said they would be," said Mr. Richardson. "And there are some differences between human milk and formula, but they don't seem as great. Now, I certainly know of some friends' children who have been raised successfully on formula. Why not? Are there differences you haven't mentioned that are more important? I remember you said something about fewer infections with breast milk. . . ."

"You are right on all counts," I said. "The differences so far between formula and breast milk are not enormous, and children have been raised successfully on formula. Now I'll tell you about the differences that cannot be corrected by the formula manufacturers—or at least they haven't been as yet. These are differences that have only recently been uncovered, differences that have very exciting implications for the nutrition of growing children.

Nutritional Immunity and Breast Milk

"Once again, we need some background. Our natural defense against disease is made up of two parts: cells in the blood which engulf infecting organisms and remove them from circulation, and certain protein molecules called antibodies or immunoglobulins produced in response to the specific type of protein in the cells of the invading germ. The three major immunoglobulins are immunoglobulins G, A, and M, and are abbreviated IgG, IgA, and IgM.

"The immune system of the baby is immature at birth. Only IgG gets to the fetus from the mother across the placenta. It provides a sort of holdover defense until the other immunoglobulins can be produced by the baby. They won't be produced, however, in sufficient quantity until the baby is two to six months old.

"Colostrum, the breast milk produced during the first three days of life, contains all three immunoglobulins. Although they are not well absorbed from the intestines of the newborn, it is known that colostrum-fed babies have greater amounts of all three in their blood than do babies not fed colostrum. The predominant immunoglobulin in colostrum and breast milk is immunoglobulin A. It is passed . . ."

"Wait a second," interrupted Mr. Richardson, who had been paying close attention throughout the discussion. "Do you mean to tell me that with modern technology and with all the other changes the pharmaceutical companies have made to

'humanize' cow's milk that they haven't been able to manufacture these immunoglobulins and add them to the formula?''

"The problem," I answered, "is that milk has to be heated
in order to sterilize it for public consumption. You've heard of
pasteurization. In the process of pasteurization these immunoglobulins, which are sensitive to heat, are inactivated.''

"And breast milk is sterile to begin with," he observed. "So
you don't need to heat it."

"That's right. There might be an occasional virus that is
passed along in the milk, but there are no bacteria. Nothing
to necessitate heat treatment if the milk is coming straight from
the breast to the baby. And there's another very elegant twist
to the story which we haven't gotten to yet."

I went on to explain that the IgA that is found in colostrum
and mature breast milk does not get absorbed from the gastrointestinal system and, as far as the otherwise poorly de-
fended infant is concerned, that may be its greatest asset. It
coats the inner lining of the digestive system from the top to
the bottom and prevents infecting germs from being absorbed.

It does this by forming a specific antigen-antibody complex
that inactivates the bacteria. The antigen is the bacteria; the
antibody is the immunoglobulin. The complex is formed when
the two come together—like two pieces that match in a jigsaw
puzzle. In order for the two pieces to match, it's best if they
have been exposed to each other in advance. In most cases,
when we get infected we develop symptoms as the bacteria
multiply. Meanwhile, the antibodies are being produced to
match the invader. Once they are produced in sufficient
amount, the invasion is thwarted and life goes on as usual.

The elegant aspect of the IgA defense is that it is already
developed to interact specifically with the bacteria that are in
the baby's environment. This is because the cells that produce
IgA in the mother originate in her intestinal tract, where they
react to the particular types of bacteria that are there. It appears that these same cells migrate through the bloodstream
of the mother to her breast tissue, where they secrete their

bacteria-specific IgA into the breast milk, or possibly where they enter the breast milk themselves.

"So that when the baby is exposed to the same bacteria as are in the mother's intestine," said Mr. Richardson, "there is no time wasted for production of the specific antibody. It's already there."

"Exactly," I said. "And the bacteria in her intestine are usually the same bacteria the baby will be exposed to."

"That's absolutely amazing," said Mrs. Richardson. "You mean my body knows enough to do all that?"

"All that, and more," I said. "You see, your breast milk also supplies the other kind of defense. There are cells called 'macrophages' in the breast milk. They engulf the germs, which are then removed from circulation.

"Remember, all of this defense material is present in fresh breast milk. Once the milk is stored at freezing temperatures or heated for pasteurization it loses these characteristics."

"What about if I want to save some of my breast milk to feed the baby later in the day?" asked Mrs. Richardson.

"You can safely refrigerate it for as long as 12 hours without any ill effects on the protective mechanisms. Just don't freeze it," I said.

"There are two other potential mechanisms," I continued, "that help in this 'nutritional immunity' of breast milk, as it is called. One of them affects the kind of bacteria that end up growing in the infant's originally sterile intestinal tract. As long as the baby drinks breast milk and *only* breast milk, there is never any growth of the bacteria which we, as adults, have in our intestines. A particular bacterium named *Escherichia coli*, usually abbreviated *E. coli*, is one of many which may be capable of causing serious diseases in the young infant. Bacteria capable of causing diseases are called pathogens. The baby has no *E. coli* in the intestines as long as the baby drinks breast milk exclusively. As soon as a supplementary bottle or solid food is added, the intestine grows over with bacteria—including *E. coli*—just like an adult's."

"Does that *always* lead to serious diseases?" asked Mr. Richardson.

"Fortunately not, but the potential for such infections is greater when the organisms are around," I said.

The other mechanism that I explained to the Richardsons involves another advantage of breast milk that at first seems separate from its ability to protect against disease: the efficient absorption of iron from breast milk. Bacteria capable of causing disease, like *E. coli,* need iron for their normal growth. One of the proteins in whey, called "lactoferrin," binds iron and helps it to be absorbed. Lactoferrin that is left over after the dietary iron has been absorbed will bind the iron which is necessary for bacterial growth, eventually leading to its inhibition. Lactoferrin is produced by the macrophage cells along with enzymes called "lysozymes," which help the IgA destroy the bacterial cell.

"Lactoferrin, then, is a whey protein, and there's more whey in breast milk than in cow's milk. None of this lactoferrin is present in infant formula?" Mrs. Richardson asked.

"None. And the end result is that infants who are raised on breast milk alone, even for the first few months, have fewer intestinal infections."

"You said something before about fewer respiratory infections as well. How does that fit in?"

"It isn't clear how. However, it seems that breast-fed babies may also have fewer respiratory infections, and there are studies in societies where breast milk is used more extensively than in ours that show a significant reduction in the number of ear infections."

"Why?"

"Why? No one knows," I admitted. "Maybe it's because germs reach the ear or the lungs by passing through the mouth where the concentration of IgA in a breast-fed baby may be sufficient to impede their progress. Or they might be prevented from entering the bloodstream because absorption in the intestines is blocked by IgA. I don't know."

"I have a friend who told me that children who breast-feed have fewer allergies later in life," said Mrs. Richardson. "Can you tell us about that?"

Prevention of Allergies and Breast Milk

"That does seem to be true. It is related to the same IgA that is important for nutritional immunity. Remember, we said it worked by forming an antigen-antibody complex with the invading bacteria. Well, the IgA is reacting to the protein part of the bacteria. And it reacts pretty much the same way to any foreign protein—that is, any protein new or unfamiliar to the body. For instance, it is capable of forming an antigen-antibody complex with the foreign protein of cow's milk, and by doing so it prevents that protein from being absorbed."

"What does cow's milk protein have to do with allergies?" asked Mr. Richardson.

"Most of the allergic reactions we experience are in response to foreign protein that gets into our bloodstream. In older children and adults, the intestines are capable of blocking large protein molecules and keeping them from being absorbed in a form that may cause an allergic reaction. Small infants have an immature intestinal wall that isn't capable of preventing those protein molecules from being absorbed. And it is suspected, but again unproved, that absorption of them leads to allergies later on in life."

"This is all very interesting. Let's see," said Mr. Richardson, as he counted on his fingers. "Breast milk is more easily digestible, has better quality protein and fat that's more easily absorbed, contains less salt and very low renal solute load, offers better defense against disease, leads possibly to fewer allergies, and . . . something about iron and lactoferrin." Mr. Richardson had been taking notes.

"Yes, something about iron and lactoferrin," I responded. "It was thought for a while that drinking breast milk would lead to iron deficiency because of its low iron content. And

when the pharmaceutical companies added iron to their formulas they had to raise the iron concentration to a level 10 to
12 times greater than that in breast milk in order to provide
sufficient iron for the growing baby's red blood cell production. This added to the fear that breast-fed babies really
weren't getting enough iron. However, when their iron levels
were measured and when someone assessed their ability to
produce red blood cells, all was found normal. The investigators concluded that the iron in breast milk, although present
in small quantities compared to that in iron-fortified formulas,
is absorbed more efficiently. And the reason this is so may be
due to the presence of lactoferrin in breast milk. Lactoferrin is
called a 'carrier protein'; it may work by picking up the iron
in the intestine and carrying it across the intestinal wall to the
bloodstream."

"Is there *any* nutrient that breast milk is deficient in?" asked
Mr. Richardson.

"If you're asking if it is necessary to supplement breast feeding with vitamins, the answer is no. But we'll go into more
detail on that later. Human milk has proved sufficient for human growth for thousands of years. One of the problems of
our civilization is that we always believe we can improve on
nature. I'm not sure this is an area where we will succeed. In
any case, there also seems to be a psychological gain in breast-
feeding—a gain that our unquestioning ancestors undoubtedly
sensed.

Mother-Child Bonding

"A gain for the baby or the mother?" asked Mrs. Richardson.

"Probably for both, but it's hard to tell about the baby. I
suspect the baby benefits as well, particularly if the breast-
feeding is started in the delivery room."

"What's the advantage of breast-feeding the new baby in
the delivery room?" Mrs. Richardson asked.

"The advantage for the baby is that it probably affords the
infant a more gentle introduction to an otherwise cold world.

After all, the mother's womb is a dark, warm, moist environment, where every stimulus the baby receives is muted. There are no shocks until birth. To take a baby from that safe environment and suddenly put the infant in dry sheets on a mattress seems unnecessarily harsh. And it was never done this way until modern times. It may just seem better, but I like the idea of a mother snuggling up with her baby and forming a substitute womb with her stomach, breasts and arms."

"It does sound nice," said Mrs. Richardson, "much better than an abrupt transition. But what are the positive effects for the mother?"

"In recent years, psychologists and pediatricians have been impressed with a phenomenon called 'mother-infant bonding.' Mothers who can hold their babies in the first twelve hours of life—and by that I mean close to them, touching them, skin to skin contact if possible—seem to satisfy their own mothering needs more. They not only say that they feel closer to their babies, but that they are more open and responsive to them as well. They experience less apprehension and fear than mothers who are kept from their babies in the first twelve hours—as many mothers are in our hospitals.

"Apparently, when a mother sees that her baby is normal right away; that it sucks, swallows, breathes on its own; that it isn't disfigured in any way but is beautiful and normal, all her anxiety is relieved. For a mother who has to wait to see her baby, the anxiety builds up. And when it builds up, the mother tends to withdraw from the baby, unconsciously probably, in order to protect herself from feeling too upset if something actually *is* wrong. Breast-feeding right after delivery lets her feel like a mother right away—she doesn't have a chance to question it. Not only that," I continued, "but it may be that 'bonding' of this nature leads to less child abuse later in the child's life."

"Do you believe all of this?"

"I tend to. Still, a lot of mothers describe the same feelings even though they weren't with their baby right away, or even if they adopted their child. All the mothers I know who have breast-fed their babies immediately describe it as an absolutely fantastic feeling. And the occasional mother whose baby was unfortunately transferred to an intensive care unit for the first days has sometimes told me she feels as if she has never had a baby at all. After all, our grandparents and great-grandparents were breast-fed early as a matter of course. It just seems to be taking us a long time to get things back to where they were."

"From what you say, there can be no question about whether to breast-feed or not. Surely the controversy wouldn't be so active if it were so unquestionably good. What are the arguments against breast-feeding?" asked Mr. Richardson.

Arguments Against Breast-Feeding

"I'll tell you what they are," said Mrs. Richardson. "That it can be painful. That it interferes with any hope the woman may have of pursuing a career. And that some of the pollutants in our environment, or any medications the mother might have to take, will be passed on to the baby."

"That just about covers all of them," I said. "I might add that it also tends to exclude the father from the feeding process, which can be a major drawback. Let's take them one at a time. We'll start with pollutants and medications in breast milk. But first a bit of background on that subject."

Drugs, Pollutants and Breast Milk

I went on to explain that this is a controversial area largely because remarkably few hard facts are known about the subject. Studies done on animals have supplied us with almost all we know about the subject, since experimenting on nursing mothers and their babies is very difficult, and in most situations would be unethical. The other problem is that not all nursing mothers are the same in what they excrete into their breast milk.

As a rule, I assume that every medication a mother takes will pass into her breast milk in some quantity. I also assume that most medications will be in such a form or in such small amount as to be insignificant to the infant. This means that the majority of infants should continue at the breast regardless of the medications taken by the mother. There are exceptions, and the exceptions are important. They occur, in general, when the mother is taking large doses of any drug, or when the drug is new on the market and its effects on the infant may not be known. Examples of drugs which are dangerous when taken in excess—and by this we mean more than the usual prescribed amount—are diazepam (Valium), ethyl alcohol, chloral hydrate, and phenobarbital. They all cause sedation in the newborn.

Nicotine is a drug which delivered to the baby in milk may cause restlessness, nausea, and vomiting. These symptoms may occur if the mother smokes more than 20 cigarettes a day. (It has been reported that smoking 20 to 30 cigarettes per day may also reduce the amount of milk produced by the mother.)

Other commonly taken drugs, such as salicylates (aspirin) and caffeine as they are commonly used—that is, for headache or to keep moving in the office—do not pose a threat to the infant. The same is apparently true for some antibiotics, such as penicillin or ampicillin. However, others, such as chloramphenicol (Chloromycetin), metronidazole (Flagyl), and the tetracyclines, are best avoided.

"What about the argument that pollutants like PCBs and DDT are passed into breast milk in an amount greater than that found in either cow's milk or formula?" asked Mrs. Richardson.

"I share your concern about this, and so do any number of concerned doctors and epidemiologists now doing work in this area. But so far there is no conclusive proof that either of these chemicals has harmed the breast-fed infant. My feeling is this: we know a lot about the benefits of breast milk on the growing infant, more than we know about the possible ill effects of these chemicals. Nothing of an extraordinary nature has become evident with regard to the latter. I will continue to recommend breast milk unless a realistic case is someday made against it."

"How can we keep all those other drugs you mentioned straight?" asked Mrs. Richardson. "Aspirin is safe, Valium may not be, don't use tetracyclines. There are so many, and I know you didn't mention all of them."

"When in doubt, consult your pediatrician. If he or she does not mention the possible effects of the drug on the breast-feeding baby, then ask about them. In almost every case, the drug can either be removed, changed to a more benign one, or reduced in amount. A mother rarely has to stop breast-feeding because of common drugs or medications."

In our discussion, Mrs. Richardson raised other issues that have frequently served to discourage the young mother from breast-feeding. In the days when breast-feeding was more prevalent, these issues would have been resolved by any one of a number of supportive figures—mother, aunt, sister, grandmother—who had breast-fed their babies. In many parts of our society today, the mother interested in breast-feeding is discouraged rather than encouraged by the experiences of other mothers, who themselves were rarely encouraged to breast-feed. In this way, myths and misconceptions rather than proper instruction have been passed from generation to generation, to the extent that a mother who today decides to try breast-feeding may actually be seen as breaking from her "heritage." When questions are raised by mothers who intend to breast-feed, the pediatrician, obstetrician, and especially the nurse must provide the necessary support in the form of education, preparation, and encouragement.

Common Questions and Answers About Breast-Feeding

We discussed Mrs. Richardson's concerns one by one. Here are her questions and my answers:

Does it ruin your figure? No. Although there is no clear evidence that support is necessary, some women who provide support for their breasts by wearing the appropriate bra feel more comfortable. Many women who have breast-fed have maintained their figures; some believe it improved their figures. The anxiety about this issue arises from the enlargement of the breast secondary to the hormonally stimulated increase in mammary tissue and the deposit of fat mentioned earlier as a store for lactational energy.

Does it always have to be messy? No. Most women find that although their breasts may leak, they can control this by using absorbent pads, and that it is essentially not a problem. The letdown of milk is controlled by a hormone called "oxytocin" that is very sensitive to emotions and can be triggered, in some cases, just by *thinking* about breast-feeding. (It can also be impeded by emotions such as fear or anxiety.) Leaking of milk from the breasts should be viewed as a totally normal hormonal response of the body. It really is not messy—and after all, it *is* sterile.

Can you keep your job and still breast-feed? Yes. But it is hard to do in our society. Some mothers express extra breast milk in the morning and leave it in a bottle for the baby's day-keeper to give the baby. Others use a supplemental bottle but find they must pump their breasts often at the beginning of lactation to keep from becoming engorged. In some enlightened working places, a nursery is available where the mother can leave her baby and return to breast-feed her every three hours or so. The point is, it can be done. A number of interns and residents of my acquaintance have had babies and continued to breast-feed after they returned to work. Their only complaint was that in addition to being tired from their very demanding jobs, breast-feeding further exhausted them for the first two months. Which raises the next question:

Is it exhausting? Yes and no. Breast-feeding takes a lot of energy, and the breast-feeding mother tends to feel exhausted, or at least a little tired, at the beginning—usually the first six to eight weeks. This is when she burns up many of the calories she put on during her pregnancy. Most mothers, however, feel "more like themselves" by the time the child is two months old. When they reach this point, they generally feel as if they could breast-feed forever.

Is it painful? Again, yes and no. There are uncomfortable times, particularly in the first week, when the breasts become engorged as the mother makes more milk than the baby needs. After that, it can definitely be clear sailing without discomfort. Some mothers get cracked nipples, which results from drying of the skin of the nipple. The condition is analogous to chapped lips in cold weather—and just as uncomfortable. But not everybody gets chapped lips, and certain preliminary measures, like massaging the nipples prenatally and smearing them with a lanolin moisturizing cream postnatally, will help prevent the problem. Also, as uncomfortable as it may sound, many mothers nurse right through this stage or at least express milk from the affected breast in order to avoid engorgement.

Do you have to start breast-feeding in the delivery room? No. But it is the best place and time to begin. It stimulates the hormone which causes milk production (called "prolactin") and the hormone which causes milk letdown (oxytocin). Oxytocin is the same hormone which stimulates uterine contraction and so helps stop postnatal uterine bleeding. There are, however, many instances of women who wished to breast-feed their babies months after birth and succeeded, even if they had not been expressing milk for that period of time. There are also mothers who have breast-fed adopted children. This is called relactation. A mother who has not breast-fed her baby in the delivery room should not be discouraged from starting later. If she was anesthetized for the delivery she will hardly be in any condition for breast-feeding in the delivery or the recovery rooms. However, the sooner the easier—and maybe the better. Indications are that it does help strengthen the bond between mother and child.

Can any woman breast-feed?   Yes.

Does it matter what size her breasts are?   No. Size of the breast has no correlation with adequate function. Milk will be produced in adequate amounts and letdown will occur at appropriate times no matter what size the breasts are. Remember, the vast majority of breast-feeding failures are caused by failure to let down the milk (often because of anxiety), *not* because of failure to make enough.

Is it true that breast-feeding excludes the father from the joys of feeding his child?   Not necessarily. He can be the one to feed the extra bottle of expressed milk, or a supplemental bottle, when the baby is just a few months older. There are other techniques for participation, like holding the baby after each feeding. The point is that the father can share in the exhilaration of nurturing his baby even though only the mother is physiologically adapted to nursing the infant. Both parents should discuss the "ground rules" of feeding, so that neither feels excluded from the process. Sharing is very possible.

"We'll talk more at length about some of these things when the time comes," I said to the Richardsons. "For now, I'll consider it a success if we've answered some questions and quieted some fears."

"What do you see as the major drawback to breast-feeding?" It was Mrs. Richardson who asked.

I leaned back and thought for a moment. "Well, I think that if *either* of the parents is not eager to do it, it won't be successful. I mean that. I really don't think one member of the couple is more important in this matter than the other. The times I've seen it fail have been when the mother felt pressured into doing it. She was made to feel that she wouldn't be a good mother if she didn't succeed at breast-feeding. Or the father merely felt resigned to putting up with it—that somehow this was something he simply had to tolerate for a couple of months. If all questions are answered satisfactorily, and one parent is still against it, then I don't think the mother should breast-feed. When one tries to do it against the other's wishes and fails, considerable guilt and anger can ensue.

I turned to Mr. Richardson. "Right now, I'd be very interested to know what you're feeling, Mr. Richardson. We seem to have been concentrating mostly on your wife's concerns."

The Father's Concerns

He responded slowly and thoughtfully. His first concern was that he was going to be excluded from a primary relationship with his new child by not feeding it. He was also worried about being excluded from his wife's attention and time, particularly if breast-feeding took as long as many of his friends had told him it would.

"How do you envision this breast-feeding occurring?" I asked.

"It'll probably be the way it was with Lucille's friend. She breast-fed every three hours or so, sometimes more frequently. She insisted on being totally alone while she did it. She said the milk wouldn't come down if she wasn't. And each feeding took a half-hour or more." He looked at me again. "I can't imagine Lucille having time for more than one relationship, if that's the case."

"Do you think it has to be like that?" I asked.

"I don't know; that's what I wanted to ask you."

Here Mrs. Richardson answered her husband. "I didn't know you felt that way at all, John. I don't plan to lock myself in a room for this. I've always imagined it as something we would share with each other. In fact, *I'm* worried about being alone."

Her husband looked at her. "Really?"

"Oh, absolutely. I've never done this before, after all. I mean, maybe if this weren't our first child I wouldn't feel so anxious, but I feel like I need all the support I can get."

We talked more about the Richardsons' fears, which they

were both open to discussing. I assured them that the hospital where Mrs. Richardson was planning to deliver did allow "rooming-in"—the baby would stay in the mother's room. This practice replaces the outmoded one of keeping the baby in the nursery and bringing her to the mother only every three hours for a feeding—a practice obviously not suitable for breast-feeding on a demand-feeding schedule. ("Demand feeding" means feeding the baby whenever she's hungry—usually every two to three hours, but maybe more frequently in the first days.)

The Richardsons made their decision to breast-feed after considering the available data and carefully weighing the pros and cons. Although I personally believe it desirable, I realize that not all parents will arrive at the same decision. Pediatricians and other doctors who are proponents of breast-feeding are most frustrated, however, when parents make their decision to bottle-feed out of ignorance, simply from not having been told about the advantages of breast-feeding. It is also frustrating when a mother begins breast-feeding and then switches immediately to the bottle because no one is available to support her through the difficult early days.

If parents do decide to bottle-feed, however, I support them completely. After all, a lot of children have been raised successfully on the bottle by parents who nurtured them well. No mother should be made to feel guilty because she does not breast-feed. She may find that her loving concern for her child is more comfortably expressed by bottle-feeding. And although it is frustrating to see someone stop breast-feeding because of lack of support, it is better to stop than to continue merely for fear of being called a bad mother or a failure. Parents who are happy with themselves provide the best environment for a child to grow in.

CHAPTER 3

The Breast and the Production of Breast Milk

ONCE THE DECISION to breast-feed has been made, prenatal preparation is enhanced by a more in-depth knowledge of the physiology and anatomy of the breast and the production of breast milk itself. Knowing how and when the milk is produced and understanding the commensurate changes in the breasts can do much to reduce anxiety and make the more difficult first days pass by more easily. Without such instruction many mothers stop breast-feeding because they are afraid that terrible things are happening to them, or that the problems they are confronting will go on forever. In addition, problems (such as breast abscesses) can arise which might have been avoided by some timely advice.

Anatomy

We can better understand the internal anatomy of the breast by studying the production and flow of human milk. The area of the breast we will concentrate on is called a lobe—the breast being made up of from 10 to 20 lobes, each containing its own milk-producing machinery.

In each lobe, milk production occurs deep in the breast in sac-like glands called "alveoli." A number of alveoli are clustered together rather like grapes. Each alveolus drains the milk secreted into it into a common branching duct—imagine the duct as the main twig holding a cluster of grapes. In each lobe there are a large number of these grape-like clusters, each drained by a branching duct. Milk flows from the clusters through the branching ducts toward the nipple. Externally the nipple is surrounded by a pigmented halo of tissue called the "areola." Under the areola each duct suddenly expands to form a large collecting reservoir into which the milk flows. The milk which is secreted in drops in the alveoli is now collected in larger volumes in these reservoirs (called the "lactiferous sinuses"). There is one reservoir for each lobe. From the reservoir milk runs out a final large duct (called the "lactiferous duct") through the nipple.

Physiology

This, then, is the form of the breast. The function of the breast is a bit more exciting. As pregnancy progresses, the breasts enlarge and the nipples and areolae get larger and more sensitive. Milk is produced in the glandular tissue of each breast and secreted into each alveolus following stimulation by a hormone (called prolactin) released from the brain. The brain releases prolactin when the breast is empty of milk. Consequently, as the baby suckles, prolactin is released and more milk is produced. After the baby has stopped feeding and the alveoli are once again allowed to fill with milk, prolactin is turned off and the body waits to produce milk until the next feeding. This system is aptly called a "feedback mechanism."

There is no reason for the milk in the alveoli simply to flow into the ducts and out the nipple. In fact, if this *were* the case the mother's breasts would be leaking constantly and prolactin-stimulated milk production would go on interminably—obviously an inefficient and expensive system.

Instead, what does happen is that milk collects in the alveoli until squeezed out by small muscle cells that surround them and the branching ducts. These muscle cells are stimulated to contract by the other hormone, oxytocin. Oxytocin is another part of the feedback system: sucking at the breast stimulates nerves which transmit a message to the brain calling for the release of oxytocin. Oxytocin causes the milk to be ejected from the alveoli and squeezed down the branching ducts to be collected in the reservoirs under the areola. The entire process is called milk "letdown." Mothers know when it happens. They can feel the milk flow into both breasts simultaneously, since sucking at one breast stimulates milk letdown in the other breast as well. However, once the baby has stopped suckling, oxytocin is suppressed and the ejection of milk ceases, allowing the alveoli to fill with milk for the next feeding.

Emotions such as anxiety and excitement can interfere with oxytocin release, which is why the mother who wishes to breast-feed should try to be in a peaceful environment during the feeding process.

The fact that the reservoirs are under the areola explains why the baby must get her mouth around that part of the breast in order to be fed—sucking on the nipple alone will not be enough. The compression of the reservoirs by the baby's tongue and the sucking action of the mouth push the milk up the final duct through the nipple and into the mouth.

The day the baby is born, the mother's entire feeding system is full of colostrum, a thin, watery fluid that contains more protein, less sugar, and considerably less fat than mature breast milk. It also contains fewer calories per ounce than mature milk. In addition, the amount of the protective immunoglobulin IgA is greater in colostrum than in mature milk, a point of particular interest when considering protection against disease in the nursery days of life.

In medieval times, it was felt that colostrum was bad for babies, probably because its consistency was so different from that of mature milk. As a result, either babies were fasted for their first three to five days, until the mature milk came in, or they were fed a gruel of flour and water called "pap." (It is also interesting that in those times babies were purged immediately after birth to rid them of what we now call retained amniotic fluid and meconium.)

The high protein content, low fat content, and increased vitamin and mineral concentration of colostrum are particularly suited to the needs of the newborn. Colostrum, however, changes gradually into transitional milk when the baby is three to five days old. Transitional milk can be thought of as nutritionally a mixture of mature milk and colostrum. Its caloric content approaches but does not quite equal the higher caloric content of mature milk. Transitional milk changes into mature milk by the time the baby is a week to ten days old.

Milk production will not be stimulated until the colostrum is expressed or suckled from the breast. Failure to suckle will inhibit milk production, and the ability to secrete milk will be significantly depressed after two to three weeks.

CHAPTER 4

Getting Started

The First Week—Breast-Feeding

Once the baby is born, theory rapidly gives way to actuality. Things happen so quickly that there is no time to "review notes" or to wonder if what is being done is the right thing to do. Given a supportive environment and parents who have given forethought to their baby's feeding, the best thing to do at this point is to trust the mother's and baby's instincts. The first feeding, sometimes approached with more concern than it warrants, is, after all, an instinctual act. Given a breast or a bottle, the baby who is not depressed from the mother's anesthesia will begin to suck and swallow by natural reflex.

Babies should certainly be fed in the first 6 to 12 hours of life. For some babies an early feeding is more important than for others. In addition to its effect on mother-infant bonding, the first feeding is important for the immediate energy it provides. At this point, the sugar contained in colostrum is more important to the baby than the protein. Sugar in the form of glucose or glycogen is the energy source of the body when it needs energy right away. Fat is a stored form of energy and will be used as a major source of energy only after the body glycogen is depleted. Protein is a very poor source of energy (as we shall see when we come to discuss nutrition and exercise in Chapter 8).

The stress of delivery can sometimes exhaust the baby's carbohydrate stores, leading to a decrease in blood sugar. This is particularly true for very small babies (under 5 pounds), very large babies (over 9 pounds), and babies who have had a particularly difficult delivery. The small babies need early sugar feedings because they do not have enough carbohydrate stores to begin with. (They generally have depleted fat stores as well.) The large babies need early feedings because the loss of heat over their large body-surface areas requires more energy expenditure in order to keep their bodies at normal temperature. Those who had difficult or prolonged deliveries have essentially been through an exhausting event—something akin to a neonatal marathon. Average-sized babies who have had average deliveries have absorbed enough sugar from the mother by way of the placenta to manage for the first twelve hours at least.

When I came to see Mrs. Richardson she was half sitting in bed with her baby, now six hours old, at her breast. She told me her husband had gone home to freshen up after being with her during labor and delivery. She looked tired but exhilarated. She told me everything had gone well, both with the labor and with the delivery, and that she had started feeding her little girl in the delivery room.

"It was so easy," she said of the feeding. "I was in tears from the absolute joy of it all. What a high! The doctor gave me the baby after the umbilical cord was cut and I put her right to the breast. She found the nipple right away and started suckling. She was wonderful!"

"It sounds like you did a wonderful job yourself," I said.

"Well everybody helped. The nurse showed me how to hold my breast so the nipple would stick out. Using the hand opposite the breast of course. I'm supposed to put my index finger above it, and press up and in a little, like this. See, it works," she said as she demonstrated.

By holding her breast in this way she was able to make a cone out of the nipple and the areola for the baby to suck on. It allowed her infant girl to form a neat airtight seal around the cone. The baby was blissfully sucking on Mrs. Richardson's left breast as I watched.

"And," Mrs. Richardson went on, "the nurse showed me how to move her from one breast to the other gently. Watch. It's just about time for a switch." She gently moved the little finger of her right hand into the corner of the baby's mouth where it was fixed to the breast. As she did so, there was a little sucking sound, not a pop, as she broke the air seal. She then easily moved the baby into her other arm. She grasped her right breast now with her left hand, nipple and areola between index and middle fingers, and gently guided the nipple to the baby's mouth. Her baby girl was moving her head, with her mouth still making some sucking movements, so the target was not an easy one. But as soon as Mrs. Richardson touched the baby's cheek near the corner of the baby's mouth with the nipple, the baby moved her mouth right to the nipple and started sucking again.

"How does she do that?" she asked. "As soon as I touch her cheek with the nipple she settles right on it."

"That's called the 'rooting reflex,' " I said. "Whenever a newborn baby is stroked on the cheek, the infant will turn the head toward the stimulus and start sucking on it, whether it's a finger or a nipple. The response to the stimulus gets stronger the closer you get to the corner of the mouth. That's the most sensitive area. It's another one of those reflexes that has obvious survival value. Given half a chance, a baby will find the breast and start to eat."

"One question I do have. . . . The nurse forgot to show me. How do I burp her? I've seen a lot of people do it different ways."

"First of all," I said, "burping is necessary because, invariably, whether you breast- or bottle-feed your baby, she'll take some air in with the food. If she gets too much air it can give her a false sense of fullness and interfere with her appetite. It might also lead to gas and crampy abdominal pains. Sometimes the air bubble is large and ready to come up as soon as baby is put in an upright position. Sometimes there are many little air bubbles mixed with the food that have to coalesce before she'll burp. Tapping *gently* on the back helps this happen. You never have to pound your baby, and you don't have to bounce her up and down. Just gently tap her back, with the baby in an upright position, preferably over your shoulder."

"What happens if she doesn't burp?" asked Mrs. Richardson.

"She may not," I answered. "Don't worry about it. It is a good idea, however, particularly if she doesn't burp, to lay her on her stomach after feeding. That way, if the bubble does come up with a little of her food on top of it, she won't gag on it. Try burping her as you change her from one breast to the other, and again at the end of the feeding."

"I was also advised," Mrs. Richardson continued, "to feed her for only five minutes at each breast to start with. Is that all?"

"It's not a bad idea to start gradually in these first few days. It's something of a conditioning period for your nipples. I recommend starting at five minutes on each breast and increasing the time by an additional minute each day. You're less likely to get cracked nipples if you toughen them gradually."

"Why does it have to be alternate breasts?" she asked.

"At first, that's so the baby can get enough colostrum without taxing one nipple too much. It also serves to empty both breasts of the colostrum evenly. Later you will want to make sure that you empty at least one breast completely—most of each feeding will be done at one breast, a different one each time. That's so that you stimulate prolactin secretion to the maximum and guarantee adequate milk production."

"You said that I'm making sure she gets enough colostrum. How much is enough? And how do I know she's getting it?"

"Babies' caloric needs at birth are not very great. Babies in the first three days need only 50 to 60 calories per kilogram of body weight per day. This means that if your little girl weighs 4 kilograms—that's roughly 8 pounds, 12 ounces—she needs 240 calories a day. By the end of the first week she'll be taking twice as much—roughly 120 calories per kilogram of body weight each day. But counting calories for babies is not necessary when they're breast-feeding. Trust their hunger instinct. They will tell you when they want to eat more. Their instinct for self-preservation is strong."

"Elizabeth—we've decided to name her Elizabeth—has been sleeping pretty much since the delivery," said Mrs. Richardson. "She wakes up and cries a little, so I give her the breast. Am I supposed to feed her every time she cries, or should I put her on a schedule?"

"Since the demands of babies in the first days are so variable, and since your milk will be changing so much in its own consistency from day to day, from feeding to feeding, and even during the feedings, you and I have no way of knowing if she is getting what she needs. Only she knows that, and she'll let us know by crying when she's hungry. At first her crying times may vary," I continued, "depending on how many calories she got from the last feeding and how active she's been in using them up. Most of her calories will go for growth, which is something we can measure carefully in the first month, but not in the first week. Eventually, as your milk and her needs become more consistent, she'll put herself on a schedule, probably with a little help from you. For now I think the best thing to do is what you're doing—feed her by demand, when she's hungry."

"You've told me she's getting colostrum now and that the transitional milk may come in any time in the next three to five days. But how will I know?"

"As the transitional milk comes in, you'll begin to get a very full feeling in your breasts. If they become too full, they will actually be painful. This is called 'engorgement.' The feeding technique the nurse taught you is very useful if your breasts become engorged—it tends to give the baby a better-shaped areola to suck on. You may have to express milk manually from your breasts when they become engorged in order to reduce the discomfort and facilitate the baby's feeding. Otherwise, engorgement may lead to a decrease in milk production."

I went on to explain that engorgement in the first days is caused more by swelling of the ducts than by milk production that exceeds the demands of the infant. This is a result of hormonal stimulation. As more milk is produced than consumed, the breasts enlarge to such a degree that the areola becomes indistinguishable in contour from the rest of the breast, which swells around the nipple. The new contour is flat, not conical, so the baby, finding it impossible to get the air seal around the areola, cannot suck efficiently and the breast cannot be drained. If this continues, in addition to the painful engorgement, the alveoli will not become drained, prolactin will be suppressed, and milk production will drop off.

Regular drainage of the breasts either manually or with a breast pump can prevent this and also two other consequences, called "caking" and "mastitis." Caking is a backing up of milk in one lobe of the breast as the swelling in adjacent lobes prevents its drainage. In some instances the flow is obstructed downstream from the alveoli so that milk continues to be produced behind the obstruction. The consequence of swelling and inflammation of that lobe of the breast is a painful condition called mastitis. Mastitis is a term signifying any nonspecific inflammation of the breast. It may be caused by a bacterial infection and may progress to a breast abscess. If it is a case of bacterial infection, antibiotic treatment will be necessary and the infected breast should not be used. The baby may need some supplemental bottles of sterile water when the mother has mastitis, since the milk produced tends to become more concentrated during the infection.

"How likely is all of this to happen?" asked Mrs. Richardson a bit apprehensively.

"The engorgement is inevitable but can occur in varying degrees," I said. "If you adequately express milk during that period, it will not be painful. And if you maintain good hygiene with your nipples, keeping them clean with normal soap and water, it is highly unlikely that you will become infected."

"You said before I could express milk manually or with a breast pump. Which do you recommend?"

"That's really up to you. Some mothers prefer manual expression of milk and do it quite well. Others find that it is uncomfortable, exhausting, and inefficient. They consider the electric breast pump superior. Use whichever works best for you."

"I know you said that weighing the baby in the first week isn't useful. How will I know if she's gaining weight if I don't weigh her?" asked Mrs. Richardson.

"Actually, she may not gain weight at all in the first week, and may in fact lose weight. All babies go through this. I guess it's because of three things: their appetites are suppressed after the delivery, they won't begin to get a higher-calorie diet until the transitional milk comes in at three to five days, and they normally lose excess water that they had retained during the pregnancy. I do know that bottle-fed babies regain birth weight before breast-fed babies do because the bottle-fed babies are getting more calories from the formula right from the beginning. The point is, the weight loss is normal. Regular weight gain can be counted on by the time the baby's a week and a half old."

"And then?" asked Mrs. Richardson.

"And then, count on her doubling her birth weight, roughly, by five months of age. We'll discuss that more when I see you in two weeks," I said.

"What should I be eating during all of this?" she asked.

"Eat according to your regular diet, but add an additional 500 calories each day. That's roughly equivalent to a peanut-butter-and-jelly sandwich. Remember, most of the calories necessary for breast-feeding are coming from the fat stores you gained during your pregnancy. Trust *your* instincts, too. If you're hungry, eat a little more. There are some things you should be sure you eat. One is milk, because of its high calcium and vitamin D content. Many doctors recommend up to a quart and a half a day. It may be skim milk if you are worried about putting on weight. And be sure to eat fruits, for their vitamin C content. The rest should be the usual meats, poultry, grains and vegetables. Vegetables also contribute to the vitamin C supply.

"Remember, you're going to feel tired for a couple of months. That's normal. Don't be discouraged by it. It won't go on forever," I said.

The pediatrician's greatest challenge in the first week of breast-feeding is to make sure a mother does not become unnecessarily disheartened and stop. The week is a crucial one: the mother is already tired from the delivery, everything is new, and many of the complications begin around the third day, just as she is preparing to go home and leave the supportive environment of the hospital. Anticipation of the problems by nurses and doctors can be very helpful in avoiding an unduly anxious attitude. And close telephone communication between the mother and the pediatrician until the next visit at two weeks is essential.

The First Week—Bottle-Feeding

So far, we've discussed the cares and concerns of the breast-feeding mother in the first week. This is not to be construed as meaning that the mother who has decided to feed her baby formula has any fewer concerns or that her anxiety may be any less important. In fact, because bottle-feeding appears, deceptively, so much less complicated than breast-feeding, doctors and nurses too often forget to address the concerns and anxieties of mothers who have decided to bottle-feed.

Many of the feeding practices we've discussed are just as applicable to the formula-fed child as to the breast-fed child. Whether a baby is to be breast- or bottle-fed, feeding should begin in the delivery room. A bottle of sugar water is an adequate substitute for colostrum, providing sufficient calories in the form of carbohydrates. The mother who can give her baby this initial feeding can enjoy the close contact so essential in mother-infant bonding. Both bottle-fed and breast-fed babies should room-in with their mothers, and feeding should be on a demand schedule.

Formula feeding can begin on day one or two of life. Most babies, whether breast- or bottle-fed, are not too interested in eating until then, anyway. Some may not become active and interested until the third day. Since most hospitals have contracts with a single pharmaceutical company which provides a common formula for the nurseries, the question of which formula to feed is usually not raised until after the baby goes home. Even then, the one the baby has been started on in the hospital is usually the one continued.

The standard infant formulas (e.g., Enfamil, Similac, SMA) are essentially the same in terms of nutritional quality for the baby. They come in a prepackaged form, which is somewhat preferable although more expensive than the powdered or concentrated form. The only risk in using the powdered form is that a mistake might be made in mixing it, causing it to be either too concentrated or too diluted. If the formula is too concentrated, the baby may become seriously dehydrated. If it is too dilute, the baby may fail to thrive. Care in following the directions written on the package will avoid both of these problems.

In developing nations and in some impoverished communities of "developed" nations, the water added to the powdered formula may be contaminated with bacteria capable of causing severe gastrointestinal disease, resulting in vomiting and diarrhea. Sterilization of impure water under such circumstances is essential. This risk of contamination is why many doctors and other health professionals are opposed to pharmaceutical companies carrying out large-scale advertising campaigns for their formulas in impoverished nations. Such campaigns tend to encourage mothers to bottle-feed rather than breast-feed in an environment in which breast-feeding may be the only economically feasible and sterile form of feeding.

In any case, "humanized" formulas, as the standardized infant formulas are sometimes referred to, are superior to whole or evaporated cow's milk because of their modified protein and fat content. All of the changes made in formulas in recent years have been designed to make them as much like breast milk as possible. However, evaporated milk and whole cow's milk are useful to the baby and provide a more economical way of feeding than formulas after the baby becomes six months old. Then, the baby's gastrointestinal tract is more mature and can deal with the less easily digestible cow's milk protein and fat.

There is often a question as to whether or not a formula should be fortified with iron. For the first four months of age in a full-term, normal baby, the answer is easy: it doesn't matter. The baby has been supplied with sufficient iron to last until it is at least four months old, at which time iron fortification of the diet becomes important. However, those who argue for early iron fortification point out that giving iron from birth will guarantee well-stocked iron stores when needed. They also argue that giving an iron-fortified formula from birth eliminates the chance of the baby's not taking to it later on. The contention that iron in the formula causes an increase of gastrointestinal problems, such as colic, constipation, and diarrhea, does not appear to be true.

As I mentioned to Mrs. Richardson, bottle-fed babies tend to regain their birth weight faster than breast-fed babies, since they are being offered consistent calories from the start (20 calories per ounce, the same as in mature breast milk). Mothers in the first week must be careful not to feed the baby more than the infant wants to eat. The compulsion to finish the bottle is unnecessary and may lead to a too-rapid increase in weight and, possibly, obesity later in life. The first week is *not* too early to begin worrying about this possibility. Feeding habits (of mother *and* child) are established early in life. An opened bottle may be safely kept refrigerated for twelve hours at least.

Just as with breast-feeding, the bottle-feeding mother should try to find a quiet place to feed the baby. Anxiety on the mother's part often gets transmitted by various subtle, nonverbal signals to the baby and may make the baby a fussy eater. With the baby cradled in mother's arms, the bottle should be offered in a tilted position with the nipple down so that there is always milk and not air in the nipple. Otherwise, the baby's stomach may fill up with air and suppress the appetite.

The techniques for burping the bottle-fed baby are the same as for the breast-fed infant. The baby is held in an upright position and gently tapped on the back. Some babies seem to take forever to burp; some babies don't burp at all, or at least not consistently. This is a quite normal variation. Some mothers believe the collapsible bottle that closes down as the baby empties it reduces the amount of air available to the baby and reduces gas. These babies still need to be burped in the middle and at the end of feeding, however, since air may get in around the nipple in the process of feeding. Once again, if a baby does not burp at all, or takes a long time to burp after feedings, it is best to lay the child on its stomach. If spitting up occurs with the burp, the child won't be likely to choke.

One difference between breast-feeding and bottle-feeding is that materials must be prepared ahead of time. Although the elaborate procedures of years gone by—sterilizing bottles and nipples, use of a sterilizing rack, and so on—are no longer essential, it is important to wash the nipple and the bottle carefully, as you would the rest of the dishes, after a meal. Make certain that the hole in the nipple gets rinsed through so that it won't get obstructed. If there is any question about the quality of the water being used, switch to sterilization.

Formula may be fed to a baby warm, at room temperature, or cold from the refrigerator. It apparently makes no difference to the baby what temperature it is, even though body temperature would seem to be more natural. In this regard, I advise parents to do whatever is convenient for them.

CHAPTER 5

Feeding Your Child: From the First Week to Six Months

By the end of the first week, the breast-fed baby is receiving mature milk from the mother. Although the problems of engorgement and mastitis can occur any time in the first two months, they are more likely to do so in the first week. After the first week, the baby's appetite is becoming more regular, and most mothers will be able to identify their babies as being fast, slow, or indifferent eaters. The period from one week to six months of age is the major milk-feeding period of infancy. When the child turns six months old, solid foods will be introduced, the child may be put on cow's milk, and the entire feeding experience will take on a new dimension.

Is My Baby Getting Enough to Eat?

Probably the most common and most anxiety-provoking issue, especially for a breast-feeding mother, is "Am I feeding my baby enough? How can I tell?" Inevitably, the mother who is breast-feeding has heard stories of someone who took her constantly crying, breast-fed baby to the doctor at two weeks and was told that the baby was failing to thrive. It is terrifying for a mother to think she might be inadvertently starving her child. If she dwells on it, her anxiety will undoubtedly interfere with her milk letdown—a nutritional example of self-fulfilling prophecy.

During the first week, weight is not a useful measure of breast milk adequacy because of the great variability in weight lost and regained in that time. Weight becomes more useful as a gauge closer to one month of age. How, then, can the mother tell how much her newborn baby is getting?

"I just want an idea," Mrs. Richardson said over the phone. And then, typically, "I'm convinced she's not getting enough to eat."

Estimating adequacy of intake for a breast-feeding baby is a far more complicated task than doing so for the formula-feeder. Breasts do not come calibrated in ounces the way bottles do, and you can't weigh them before and after each feeding. You could, of course, weigh the child before and after each feeding to see how many ounces have been gained. But if worry about intake adequacy is carried to this extreme, it may create more anxiety than it calms. However, I have occasionally asked a mother who was convinced she was not producing enough milk to measure pre- and postfeeding weights (assuming she had the appropriate scales at home) for two days, just to show her that her milk supply is adequate.

A better way to gauge the adequacy of breast-feeding is to ask how long the baby takes to feed and how frequently the baby asks to be fed. The average healthy baby takes less than ten minutes to drink up 80 percent of the milk supply of one breast, with the major portion of the milk consumed in the first five minutes. As the milk is being let down during each feeding, it changes in quality. The amount of fat it contains increases. Perhaps this is a signal to the baby that the meal is finished, the fat having given more fullness to the baby's stomach. Most babies will continue to suck even when the breast is dry—presumably to answer their oral needs. This is referred to as non-nutritive suckling and is, in a sense, somewhat the equivalent of giving the bottle-feeding baby a pacifier. Mothers can frequently tell when their baby is suckling milk or when the infant is just suckling.

Mothers can also describe to their physicians how frequently their baby asks to be fed and, when offered the nipple, how the child takes to it. Average time between feedings—with a fairly wide range of what would be considered normal—is every two to three hours. For instance:

He eats like crazy for five to ten minutes on one breast then for about five minutes on the other breast, then he sort of sucks on and off at the nipple half asleep. I put him down after ten minutes or so, and he sleeps. Maybe two hours later, sometimes three at night, he starts to cry. I let him cry a couple of minutes just to be sure he means it, then pick him up and feed him again. I start with the same breast he left off from.

This should be considered absolutely normal behavior. Another example:

She's not an aggressive eater, doctor. I put her to the breast and she sucks at it somewhat continuously for, oh, ten, fifteen, maybe twenty minutes. She seems more interested in looking at my face. When she's done, I try her on the other breast but she's really not interested, so I give her that one first thing next time. When is next time? Three and a half hours—and she sleeps through the night.

This is another example of a normal feeding pattern. However, the next example is not:

She's always hungry and she cries a lot, a really colicky baby. Sometimes it drives me crazy how much she cries. I give her the breast and she starts eating like she's starved. I mean really. She sucks for fifteen minutes, sometimes more, and then on the other breast for a little. I put her down after the feeding and she sleeps, but I've hardly turned around, an hour and a half, occasionally two, and she's crying again. I let her cry because I don't want to spoil her, but when I'm ready to feed her again she's so upset she can hardly eat.

This may, in fact, be a colicky baby, but the evidence points more to a child who is not getting enough to eat with each feeding. She's always hungry, she sucks vigorously when she gets the chance, she stays long enough at the breast to drain every last drop of available milk, she's hungry more frequently than every two to three hours. There are two other ominous signs that suggest that this problem will go on unless someone intervenes: the mother is anxious because of all the crying (which came first, the anxiety or the crying, is no longer important), and the baby gets so upset she can hardly eat well when she finally gets the chance. The diagnosis will be confirmed if the baby fails to gain weight. The resolution might be to quiet the mother down by quieting the baby down. Feed the child every hour and a half, or even every hour, for a while, until her hunger is more manageable and she's less fretful. The length of time between feedings can be gradually increased as both baby and mother begin to feel more relaxed.

Here is an example of another, slightly different, abnormal situation:

He's a very picky eater, and is sort of hungry but sort of not. When he gets a chance to eat, he starts in like they're closing the kitchen in five minutes, only he doesn't even make it to five minutes: a couple of minutes . . . pooped. He sleeps. I nudge him a little with the nipple and maybe he eats a little more, but not much, even when I try him on the other breast. So I let him sleep after trying to get him to eat for a half-hour. He doesn't sleep a half-hour, and he's hungry again. I spend my whole day feeding him.

There is a different situation here than in the previous example. This baby's wanting to eat every half-hour tells us he knows he's not getting enough with each feeding. But in this case it's not because the food isn't there, it's because the baby becomes rapidly exhausted trying to eat it. This is the clinical picture of a child in marginal heart failure who has congenital heart disease or, possibly, chronic lung disease. An adult with emphysema or a heart condition will get short-winded climbing stairs or going for a walk. A baby with these diseases can show fatigue only when eating. That's the most work the infant does all day.

There are some additional points of interest in the first two examples of normal feeding behavior. The first is that the mothers alternate the breasts that they start the baby on. This assures that at least one breast is totally emptied each feeding and that prolactin is induced to stimulate maximum milk production. It is not necessary to empty both breasts for prolactin stimulation to occur. The mechanism is sensitive enough that if the baby has a small appetite or eats small quantities more frequently, less milk will be drained from the breast, less prolactin released, and less milk produced—just enough to satisfy the appetite and feeding pattern of the child.

Another point of interest is that in both examples the babies are alert and attentive to their surroundings. Babies who are actively eating *usually* do not fall asleep during the feed. They can, however, and still be normal.

One mother speaks of her child waking to be fed through the night. The other says her baby sleeps through the night. Both are normal occurrences. No two babies are exactly alike in their schedules. There are some babies who are thoroughly content, almost from the first week, to sleep throughout the night. Others will wake regularly for the 2:00 A.M., 5:00 A.M. and 8:00 A.M. feedings, and this may go on until three or four months of age. This variability occurs regardless of breastfeeding or bottle-feeding, and is unaffected by the early addition of solid foods. Unfortunately, a mother sometimes yields to frustration and begins solid foods at roughly the same age she thinks the baby should be sleeping through the night.

Finally, the parent in our first example mentions letting her child cry a couple of minutes before picking him up to feed him, just to make sure he means it. She wants to make sure it's hunger that is making him cry. How long you let a baby cry before picking him up is a point of no little controversy and depends a lot on the psychological outlook of *both* parents.

Some doctors (and parents) feel strongly that you cannot "spoil" a child under three months old by picking him up whenever he cries. (By "spoiling" they mean giving the infant positive reinforcement for crying so that he learns that crying will always result in getting picked up and held.) Other doctors (and parents) swear this is not so, that they've seen any number of children who learned before three months that they could manipulate their parents' behavior by crying.

Let me begin by acknowledging that hearing a baby cry for more than five minutes (particularly when it's your own) is very unnerving. And let me acknowledge that I have not yet learned the difference between the sound of a hungry cry and a "spoil-me" cry. I think, however, that the timing of the cry, particularly when the child has been on a more or less regular feeding schedule, can help determine its significance.

The first postnatal visit to the pediatrician is well timed at two weeks to a month. The mother has had time to get accustomed to her baby and will undoubtedly have a lot of questions ready to ask—especially the mother who may feel awkward calling the doctor with questions beforehand. Having the first visit at two weeks guarantees that the baby's nutrition will be assessed early on and that mothers will have their questions answered early so that no problems get out of hand.

"Is she growing?" asked Mrs. Richardson after I had finished weighing Elizabeth during the first postnatal visit.

"She's on her way," I said, satisfied that she had already regained and even slightly surpassed her birth weight. "We'll weigh her each time she comes into the office, without any clothes or diapers on, on the same scale. If I don't think she's growing fast enough, I'll tell you. We won't weigh her more than once a month or once every two months. Otherwise the normal day-to-day variations in weight can be confusing and anxiety-provoking." I then gave Mrs. Richardson a copy of a growth chart. "If you want to, you can take this growth chart and plot out Elizabeth's measurements at home. The growth chart will probably tell us more than anything else about your baby's normal nutrition. We can tell by any variations from Elizabeth's normal, expected growth curve whether she's eating too much or too little.''

The Growth Chart

A growth chart (see Appendix 1, pages 225–236) is a graph of the measured growth of approximately 1,000 randomly selected, normal children at different ages. The object of the chart is to indicate the range of variability of growth that still falls within the range of normal.

On the growth chart, *age* is marked along the horizontal axis and *weight, height* or *head circumference* along the vertical axis. The curved lines are labeled 95th to 5th and represent percentiles of normal children: the 95th percentile line at any age means that 95 percent of normal children at that age fall below that point (and only 5 percent above it). The 5th percentile line indicates that only 5 percent of normal children at that age are below that point, which means that 95 percent are above it.

For example: at two weeks of age Mrs. Richardson's little girl weighed 7 pounds. To chart this weight, we first locate the two-week age line halfway between the zero and the line for one month. We then make a vertical line up from that point to a point next to the mark for 7 pounds. Making a point on the graph places Elizabeth between two of the curved lines— one marked 25th and the other 50th. That means that she is in roughly the *40th percentile for weight* at two weeks of age: she is heavier than 40 percent of other children her age and lighter than 60 percent of the children her age.

The same procedure can be followed for height and for head circumference, both of which are equally important but impart different information about level and adequacy of nutrition. For the normal child, height and head circumference should be close to the same percentile as the weight—although this is not invariably the case, not even in normal, very healthy children.

Before going further, let's try to define "normal." Technically speaking, "normal" applies to any child who is growing well and is healthy. In general, we apply the term loosely to mean *average*. For instance, on the growth chart the 50th percentile—that point where half the children at a certain age weigh more and half less—does not represent *normal* weight. It represents only an average. The 95th percentile is as normal as the 5th percentile, as long as the children whose weights fall on those lines are growing well and are healthy.

Our consideration of "normal" must also take into account something called "growth rate," or "growth velocity." This rate can be approximated on the growth chart by measuring the child's growth over a few months. For example, if you were to connect all of the points on the graph that correspond to the weight of 50 percent of the children at different ages, you would arrive at the 50th percentile growth curve. In a rough way, we can make a prediction as to how much a child who is in the 50th percentile for weight at one month of age should grow in the next month, two months, six months, a year, and so on. We do this by looking ahead on the 50th percentile line and seeing what weight the baby should be at those ages.

Let us take Elizabeth Richardson as an example. If she continues to grow at the same rate as a large number of other normal 25 to 50 percentile children grow, she should be roughly 14 pounds at five months, which is approximately twice her birth weight. We can also tell just by looking at how steep the graph is in the beginning that babies grow fastest in the first three months (*approximately* 1 to 2 pounds a month) and somewhat less rapidly after six months (*approximately* 1 pound a month). We can also see that babies do in fact double their birth weight by five months, and will be close to three times their birth weight by a year.

"That isn't invariably true, is it?" asked Mrs. Richardson, who had been listening to me explain the growth chart.

"No, not by any means," I answered. "Those numbers are simply average numbers. Babies who are larger at birth grow more slowly on the average than babies who start very small. One thing to take note of is if Elizabeth's rate of growth slows down from the average for kids her size. That can be a sign of something needing attention. We would see it on her growth chart. If she were to go from, say, the 80th percentile line to the 60th percentile line, we might have to investigate the cause. 'Falling off the growth curve,' as this is called, may represent failure to thrive if the tendency persists beyond one or two months."

"Are there equal landmarks for growth in height?"

"There are, but please remember these are only estimates of what is normal or average. We use them just so we can rapidly identify the child who clearly deviates from the average."

"I understand," said Mrs. Richardson.

"As you can see from the growth chart," I said, "50 percent of children are around 20 inches at birth. They grow 9 to 10 inches in the first year, 5 inches in the second year, and 2.5 inches per year from two years until puberty. Just remember, we will do all the measurements here, and then plot them out on your growth chart and my growth chart. Measuring weight every one to two months is more than enough, since more frequent measures are easily affected by daily variations. Height, on the other hand, does not vary as much from day to day. The progress of growth in height should be relatively steady and unaffected by daily or weekly diets—or by occasional bouts of diarrhea, the way weight is. If Elizabeth takes a sudden jump in height, or a sudden plunge, it's likely it will be because we didn't measure her accurately either that time or the time before. But be sure to bring it to my attention."

Vitamins and Minerals

"When we first talked about breast-feeding," said Mrs. Richardson, "you said that my breast milk would provide all the nutrients that the baby needed and that I would not need to give her vitamins. Are you sure? My mother nearly died when she heard that you weren't giving Elizabeth vitamins. To her that's unthinkable!"

"I realize that parents are always under pressure from friends and family members when it comes to raising children," I responded, "and perhaps I owe you and your mother a more extensive explanation. After all, we may complain when our parents and grandparents intervene, particularly when they are opposed to something we feel comfortable doing. But we can't forget how useful their experience in raising children can be. The irony is that your grandmother would probably be more understanding about not giving Elizabeth vitamins than your mother. After all, manufactured vitamins did not come into use until the 1930s, and then, as with other medical discoveries, they were seen as cure-all's. We must remember that for thousands of years children were brought up without vitamin supplements."

"And some got rickets and scurvy though, didn't they?" asked Mrs. Richardson.

"Yes. Some did. But those were selective vitamin deficiencies and occurred as a result of an imbalance in the diet. Rickets occurred in children being breast-fed by mothers who were themselves deficient in vitamin D. It still occurs in such cases. Or it occurred, in rainy climates, in older children who were brought up mainly on cow's milk. Remember, milk itself is *not* naturally fortified with that vitamin. But you eat eggs, and there's vitamin D in egg yolk. You drink a quart and a half of milk per day, and milk has vitamin D. And you go out in the sun, which causes your body to manufacture its own vitamin D even if you don't eat enough. There is no possibility you could be deficient in vitamin D. Since there is enough vitamin D in your breast milk to answer your baby's daily needs, there is no possibility, either, that Elizabeth could be deficient in the vitamin."

I went on to explain that until recently this transfer of the vitamin was not believed to be sufficient. For years, in assessing the amount of vitamin D in breast milk, scientists measured only that portion that was dissolved in breast milk fat, and that portion was found to be insufficient for daily needs. Investigators in England, however, recently discovered another portion of vitamin D. This portion was dissolved in the water part of the breast milk, a part that had not been measured before, since vitamin D is one of the fat-soluble vitamins. Water-soluble vitamin D has been shown to have antirachitic properties when given to animals. ("Antirachitic" means it is capable of preventing or treating vitamin D deficiency rickets.) The water-soluble vitamin D and the fat-soluble vitamin D in breast milk have been found to provide sufficient vitamin D to answer the baby's daily requirements. Also, mothers should not be afraid to take their babies out in the sun, with due precautions of course, even in the first six months. As noted above, vitamin D is also formed by the action of the sun's rays on the outer layers of the skin.

"The other condition you mentioned, scurvy," said to Mrs. Richardson, "is a disease caused by deficiency of vitamin C. It was first seen in sailors in the days when transoceanic voyages, under sail alone, took months or even years. Scarcity of fresh fruits or vegetables, both of which are rich in vitamin C, led to the deficiency state. Scurvy may be found today but is usually related to unusual diets or to extreme malnutrition. Also, there have been occasional reports of infants breast-fed by a mother whose diet was solely brown rice and tea, *without* lemon, who developed scurvy. Vitamin C will appear in the mother's breast milk as long as the mother remembers to eat fruits and vegetables and drink fruit juices.

"The same is true for the other vitamins, vitamin A, the B vitamins, vitamin E; they're all there in your diet," I said to Mrs. Richardson, "and in your breast milk."

"Would I have had to be more careful if I had decided to formula-feed Elizabeth?" she asked.

"Ironically, even less so. The pharmaceutical companies have

done an excellent job in fortifying their formula with the necessary vitamins and minerals to match them with the recommended daily allowances of each. In either case, Elizabeth
would be getting a balanced meal."

"You mentioned vitamins and minerals. What other minerals are important besides iron? I remember your convincing
argument that breast milk has sufficient available iron."

"All of the minerals are important, so far as we know. It's
just that sometimes we don't know how important they are
until we discover a disease caused by an isolated and measurable deficiency. For instance, children who were placed on total intravenous alimentation—that means they were fed their
entire diet through a needle in their vein—whose diet was
mixed up ahead of time in a liquid form started to develop
skin lesions, showed a drop-off in their growth velocity, and
lost their appetite because their taste was impaired. They were
found, after careful review of their intravenous diets, to be
deficient in zinc. Some other children were found to be zinc
deficient and to fail to grow when they were fed a formula
low in zinc. Since 1975, when this was discovered, all formulas
have been fortified with zinc. Since the year one, however,
zinc has been very plentiful in human colostrum and remains
so in breast milk, particularly for the first two months or so.
As a matter of fact, zinc absorption served as the original model
that led to the understanding of iron absorption. You remember my telling you that iron is more efficiently absorbed from
human milk, probably because of a carrier protein which fa-
cilitates its uptake in the baby's intestines? Well, an absorp-
tion-improving carrier protein secreted by the pancreas is
known to improve zinc absorption. It was recognition of this
fact that led investigators to look for a similar carrier for iron."

"Is there any *harm* in giving Elizabeth supplemental vitamins?" Mrs. Richardson asked.

"There have been sporadic cases of vitamin A toxicity, and
a whole epidemic of vitamin D toxicity, reported in the literature. The latter occurred some twenty or thirty years ago in

England and was believed to be associated with overfortification of an infant formula with vitamin D. It caused an elevation in the serum calcium levels of the infants involved. As soon as the vitamin D was reduced in the formula, the disease disappeared. There was recently a report in the pediatric literature of two infants breast-fed for three months and then fed 2-percent-fat cow's milk, given vitamin A supplements from one month of age, fruit and yellow vegetables from two months, and two servings of chicken livers, which are high in vitamin A, daily from three months until seven months—at which time they showed signs of increased pressure inside their heads, irritability, and vomiting. When the supplementary sources of vitamin A were withdrawn, the symptoms compatible with vitamin A toxicity ceased.

"Granted, these cases are isolated and extreme. But they do point out that vitamins are not necessarily benign. If given in very high quantities over a prolonged period of time, they might be very dangerous. They are also expensive and represent just another unnecessary bottle of pills to have lying around the house. This is another area where we do not have to improve on nature."

"So I don't have to supplement my breast milk with vitamins. Do I have to supplement my milk with formula or water?"

Supplemental Feedings

"Formula, no. Water, only if she wants it, and then only one or two bottles a day will be enough. The problem with adding formula in the first two months is that it can change the bacteria that grow in the bowel, as we mentioned before. This may not necessarily be bad, but it does seem counter to a beneficial effect achieved by feeding breast milk alone.

"I perhaps should not be so dogmatic about saying no to supplemental formula. I've seen it work in more than one instance in which a mother was anxious about producing enough breast milk and, as a result, was not letting-down enough.

When she added a supplemental bottle her whole outlook on breast-feeding changed. She relaxed because she realized she was no longer burdened with *having* to breast-feed her baby. It became a pleasure, and a success.

"Many mothers, however, wait until two months to add a supplemental bottle. This allows their breasts to get maximum stimulation for good milk production and good flow by the baby's hungry sucking. After all, if the baby is being fed one meal each day by bottle, that means less drainage of the breast and less stimulation of milk production. It is also true that some babies may prefer suckling on the bottle, and they might have a difficult time staying interested in the breast. Bottle-feeding is less work than breast-feeding for the baby.

"Mothers who start supplementing after two months can be sure that the baby is now more immunologically equipped to face the world and that their milk production is now stable and sufficient. Also, such mothers are frequently going back to work and find the supplemental bottle an easier way of leaving food for their baby than expressing milk by hand for the day. Or perhaps they feel they want the baby to become accustomed to the bottle in case they can't breast-feed, for some reason."

"Like what?" asked Mrs. Richardson.

"Well, they might become ill and breast-feeding may be too exhausting."

"One of the reasons I asked about supplements," said Mrs. Richardson, "was that my husband wanted to feed the baby."

"He still can," I said, "even without supplements. Just express some milk, refrigerate it, and let him feed the baby that. He shouldn't, however," I added, "*always* be given the responsibility of the 2:00 A.M. feeding."

"No," she laughed. "We've already discussed that."

"As for water," I went on, "your breast milk has enough water in it for the baby, and so do the commercial formulas. Most babies aren't interested in water, unless maybe they are unusually thirsty in the summertime. Some kids will take sugar water, but I don't recommend it. Since they don't really need water, they certainly don't need sugar water. And it sets up bad habits for later when they have teeth."

"You said only one or two bottles of water a day would be enough?"

"Sure. But don't forget, if babies take water just before a meal they won't feel very hungry for the milk. If you're giving water to Elizabeth, and if she'll take it, do it between meals.

"There have been incidents of babies getting extremely sick when they have had nothing but water to drink or if their diet has been mainly water and only a couple of ounces of milk over a twenty-four-hour period. The sickness is called 'water intoxication.' It has the same end result as not having enough sodium in the blood. All the water goes into the brain and causes it to swell, causing headaches, convulsions, and even coma and death. But don't be alarmed. These are rare and extreme cases. It isn't going to happen with your baby."

"It won't," said Mrs. Richardson. "When did you say I would start to feel more energy with the breast-feeding?"

"Maybe another six weeks, when the baby is two months old. You are resilient, however, and doing very well. You might start feeling energetic sooner."

Between two months and four months, feeding babies becomes a daily routine. There are some changes in the infant's sleeping habits, usually seen after three months, when the baby begins to sleep through the night. Some mothers become concerned about this and ask if they should awaken their baby to make sure the child eats. As a rule this is not necessary. Babies eat when they are hungry. When they begin to miss the 2:00 A.M. feeding, they usually drink more the following morning. This is the beginning of a regular routine that will eventually culminate in "three meals a day"—but not yet. The baby still needs to be fed every three or four hours.

Some mothers may feel slightly engorged in the morning after the baby sleeps all night. Their bodies have been making more milk to compensate for the baby's increased morning appetite, and they may need to express a bit before starting the feeding.

Developmental Changes in the Child

Things may seem relatively stable on the nutritional front during this period, but in all other respects the baby is changing at a breathtaking rate. At birth, the baby is flexed up in a little ball, sleeps twenty hours a day, and can't even lift his head. At four months the infant reaches; smiles; rolls over; lifts his head, shoulders, and chest up; and looks around at the world. By six months the changes are even more striking: the baby supports not only his head but his trunk as well. He sits without help, holds on to toys and passes them from one hand to the other, and when you give him a cracker he puts it in his mouth.

We say a baby "learned" this or that trick at five months of age. But the baby has not "learned" the trick in the true sense of acquisition of knowledge. The infant has a new skill that has come solely from maturation of the central nervous system: the brain becomes more complex as the child grows older and is able to perform more complicated acts.

For instance, a child doesn't sit because instructed to do so. He sits when the parts of the nervous system that control balance are developed—first the head and neck, and then the trunk. And when the infant first does it, he doesn't do it well. He's perched in a "seated" position leaning forward with his hands on the floor between his knees. Mother holds him delicately until he seems balanced—rather like trying to balance a chair on three legs—releases him for a second, long enough to say something like "Look, he's sitting!" and then he keels over to one side. The same procedure is tried again and again, until he can do it well—normally a week or so later. By this time he's ready to sit because his brain is older, not because he finally learned his lesson. The fact that he could not do it sooner does not mean that he is stupid or slow. It just means that that part of his brain that controls sitting had not yet developed. Finally, maybe two or three weeks after this primary "tripod" sitting experience, mother pulls his hands up from between his legs and holds him sitting upright. She balances him very carefully, and then lets go. He totters, leans forward a little, overcorrects himself, leans back too far, and falls over. It wasn't for long, but he *was* sitting without support for three or four seconds, which is at least three seconds longer than he was able to two weeks earlier. And so his development continues.

Introduction of Solids: A Developmental Approach

The normal neurological development that occurs in the first six months of life is important to the baby's feeding, particularly as it relates to that perennial question: when do I start the baby on solid food? Solid foods are foods that should be fed to the baby on a spoon. Cereals, fruits, vegetables—all of the blenderized baby foods come under the heading of solid foods. And because they are fed to the baby by spoon (*not* mixed in with the bottle of milk), eating them requires a certain degree of neurological coordination. This very important fact is often misunderstood. In addition to the nutritional reasons for not adding solid foods to the diet before four months, there are developmental reasons why the baby will not be ready for them until that age.

"Why should I wait until four months?" Mrs. Richardson asked me one day when Elizabeth was a little older than two months. "A lot of my friends who have small children started them on solids by four weeks."

The simplest answer for Mrs. Richardson was that solid foods weren't necessary. Her baby was a happy, thriving child on breast milk alone. Nor was her child an exception. All babies, breast- or bottle-fed, receive adequate calories, protein, fats, vitamins, and minerals, including iron, from the breast or the formula. Our ancestors rarely started feeding solids early. To quote a classic eighteenth-century text on child rearing: "If nature ever intended us to destroy the animals around us for prey, surely we may conclude this food never could be designed for our use until such time as we had teeth to eat it." (*Letters to Married Women*, by H. Smith, 1777.) The foremost pediatric textbook published at the end of the nineteenth century states that "the majority of infants are given solid food too early and in too large quantities. Most of the attacks of indigestion during the second year are directly traceable to such gross dietetic errors." (*Diseases of Infancy and Childhood*, by Emmet Holt; Appleton & Co., 1898.) Why, then, if history speaks so strongly against the early introduction of solid foods, do we find them entering the diet at six weeks, four weeks, and even two weeks of age?

Availability is the first and most obvious answer. Modern blenderized baby foods can be eaten by anyone, with or without teeth, and the fact that they are blenderized, prepackaged, and ready to use makes them tantalizingly simple to administer to the baby.

Here are some other reasons often given for introducing solid foods early, along with my responses to them:

I started him on cereal so he would sleep through the night. The milk just wasn't holding him.

Milk and cereal both stay in the stomach roughly for the same length of time (two hours and forty-five minutes), so one is no more likely to give the child a feeling of stomach fullness than the other. Cereal mixed with water has the same number of calories as an equal volume of breast milk. Mixed with milk, it provides more calories. If the child needs more calories, he should be fed more milk. If he doesn't need more, he shouldn't take them. Overfeeding may lead to obesity later in life. Most children will stop eating when their calorie needs are satisfied. The reason many children begin to sleep through the night when their parents feed them cereal is that they are at a developmental age (usually three months) at which they are ready to do so anyway.

I was afraid that he wasn't growing well, so I started him on food.

The same argument regarding caloric intake applies here. Strained cereals (as opposed to "junior foods"), fruits, and vegetables have the same or slightly fewer calories than breast milk unless mixed with milk. It is interesting that most mothers who are breast-feeding will not mix cow's or any other milk with the strained foods. This may explain why they tend to start their babies on solid foods later than mothers who bottle-feed their babies. If babies younger than four to six months need more calories, they should be given more milk. Adding solid foods is usually overfeeding. Although it may make a child grow more, it won't make the child grow properly.

She must get so bored with just that drab milk. I wanted to offer her some food that was more varied.

In this case it is not the baby who is getting bored with the drab milk, but the mother. Babies don't stop drinking milk because they are bored with it. Indeed, when the time comes to add solid foods, they frequently take a while to get used to them since they like milk much better. But it is more fun to feed cereals and strained foods than milk—at least at first. This parent and the one in the example before seem to feel that milk isn't really food. Food comes on a spoon or a fork, and the child who eats it that way is certainly seen as growing up, more advanced than the one who doesn't. Which brings up this last example:

Mary started her baby on solids at four weeks. My baby is every bit as advanced as hers.

The early introduction of solid foods has somehow become something of a developmental landmark for some parents. Some parents refer to it with the same competitive pride as they do to their child's ability to sit early or to walk early. First of all, these early developmental "landmarks" have no real significance. Because certain children can sit before other children their age, or walk earlier, does not mean they are going to be smarter or more athletic than their peers. By the time they have all completed their developmental growth they may not be equal in their mental and physical abilities, but these early so-called landmarks are in no way indicative of which children will be better than the others.

There are good reasons for waiting until the child has developed sufficiently before offering solids. The normal action of the tongue of a suckling infant (one less than four months old) is to push up, squeezing the nipple against the roof of the mouth and then *forward*, which effectively puts pressure on the milk reservoirs at the base of the nipple. It also forms the airtight seal around the nipple at the same time that suction is being applied by swallowing. This forward thrust of the tongue is referred to as an "extrusor reflex" and can be seen whenever the nipple is suddenly plucked from the baby's mouth—the infant goes on making mouthing movements as if there were a nipple there, and can be seen sticking the tongue out with each movement. This entire process is carefully coordinated (one of the few coordinated acts a new baby performs) and is obviously designed for nipple feeding.

You can imagine what happens when mother puts a spoonful of soft mush into the mechanism. The tongue squeezes it against the roof of the mouth and then thrusts it forward and *out*, since there is no suction without a nipple. The response of the parent is either to clean the mush off baby's chin and try again, or to say baby doesn't like it and go on to the next jar. Alternatively, a mother may decide to put the food in the bottle with the milk and cut a larger hole in the nipple to make sure the baby takes it. This is not advisable for two reasons: (1) the best way to have a baby choke is to have more food coming into the infant's mouth than the infant can handle; (2) as the baby eats faster to keep up with the larger amount being delivered, he overfeeds and vomits, or eventually becomes obese because he consumes food at a rate faster than his normal appetite calls for.

As to developmental signs that a baby is ready for solid foods, think of it this way: You wouldn't eat cereal lying on your back, and neither should your baby. Wait till he has the muscle strength and coordination to be able to hold his head up, which means he should just about be able to sit on his own. That's five to six months of age.

In order to respect the baby's likes and dislikes, wait until the baby is old enough to express his needs. Pushing food out with the tongue is not an expression of dislike or of fullness. It is just a reflex, one that will disappear with time. When the baby is at an age to start solid foods, he will be able to turn his head or reach out his hand when he doesn't want any more, a skill not acquired before four months.

Other reasons for not starting solid foods at an early age are similar to those for using breast milk instead of bottle milk. The immature intestinal wall of the young infant is incapable of screening out the larger, more complex molecules that come with solid foods and that may lead to allergic reactions. Starting solid foods later increases the likelihood of a child's tolerating them well. Six months is fine for most vegetables, cereals (especially rice, but not wheat), and fruits. Meats and egg whites should be held until even later, since the proteins contained in them are the most difficult to digest.

Another reason, also considered in our discussion of breast versus bottle, is that solid foods significantly increase the renal solute load in children and may contribute to a chronically dehydrated state. The increased renal solute load may also make those children who start solid foods early less capable of tolerating a diarrheal disease.

It should also be mentioned that feeding a baby strained and junior foods is an added expense—an unnecessary one which a larger family (or many small ones, today) may find hard to support.

Indeed, some mothers are now asking why solid foods need be started before a year, particularly since they do cost so much. The answer is that babies are more receptive to new tastes and textures if they are started at six months instead of waiting until a year. Also, the iron-fortified cereals provide a healthy boost to the iron stores provided by the breast milk and by the fortified formula.

The discussion of when to start solid foods is essentially the final nutritional topic of the first six months of a baby's life. At this point, both parents deserve a pat on the back, whether the mother has been feeding breast milk or formula to her baby. If breast-feeding, the mother has survived engorgement, maybe a painfully cracked nipple, and the fatigue of the first few months. If bottle-feeding or breast-feeding, both parents have managed to cope with an appetite that is not always predictable, at times that are not always convenient. The baby is now enjoying a more regular schedule of feeding. The routine is established. Mother and father have nurtured their child through the most difficult months of infant feeding.

CHAPTER 6

Feeding Your Child:
From Six Months to One Year

MILK CONTINUES TO BE the essential element of the baby's diet in the second half of the first year, and the solid foods that are given along with milk should be seen as supplemental, particularly during the months of their introduction. Let us assume that the baby starts getting solid foods when he is six months old.

The commercial foods available are cereals with and without fruit, strained juices, vegetables, meats, and desserts. (There is also home-prepared blenderized food, which will be discussed separately.) Each will be discussed in the order of its presentation to the infant.

"Well?" Mrs. Richardson asked when I saw her baby for her six-month visit. "What do I start with first? I know it's supposed to be cereal, but I went to the store and there was rice cereal, oatmeal, mixed cereal, barley cereal, high protein, cereal with fruit and without, and I'm sure there were others. I thought you said the difficult months were over?"

Types of Solids

"Don't be discouraged," I assured her. "It's easier than it looks. Just start with dry rice cereal, no fruit. It causes a lot fewer allergies than wheat cereal and it's just as good for the baby. It contains added calcium, some of the B vitamins, and iron. That's all she really needs for now. Take it home, dilute it approximately one part cereal to six parts of water or milk."

"Milk or water? What's the difference?"

"Calories," I said. "The one diluted with milk obviously has more. I prefer diluting it with water, particularly if the water is fluoridated. It becomes an added source of fluoride for the baby's developing teeth. Also, adding cow's milk may cause an allergic reaction, which you wouldn't be able to distinguish from a reaction to the rice cereal. However, the main reason we're starting with rice cereal," I continued, "is that it is iron fortified and less likely to cause allergies."

"Why not the high protein?"

"Elizabeth doesn't need high protein, and it's not as well tolerated. And," I added, in anticipation of her next question, "cereals with fruit can be added later, once we know that Elizabeth is tolerating cereals and fruits separately, and once we're sure that she is eating other foods high in iron. Some of the cereals with fruit have less iron than the dry cereals served with water *or* milk."

"How much of it does she have to take?" she asked.

"She doesn't have to take any of it at the beginning," I said. "Remember, your breast milk is giving her everything she needs. The main reason we're starting now is so she can get used to eating a food with a new taste and texture and to eating from a spoon. This is important to keep in mind. Relax as you're feeding her—it should be fun, not a battle. Try her with a little bit at the end of a spoon. She may look a little surprised when she first tries it. That's usually worth a laugh. Try some more. If she violently objects to being fed that way, stop. Try again in a couple of days. With persistence, she'll get to like it. If you force it on her, she'll end up reacting to the forcing rather than to the food on the spoon. As you know, a six-month-old already has a personality of her own.

"There are two other things to remember as you introduce Elizabeth to solid foods: introduce only one food at a time, and let five to seven days go by before starting a new food."

The reasons for these suggestions to Mrs. Richardson have already been implied. Foods can sometimes cause an allergic reaction as the baby reacts to, usually, the new protein part of the food. An allergic reaction to food can cause a baffling array of symptoms, some of which may not be true "allergic" reactions but something akin to indigestion, infection, and so on. To associate a symptom with a food definitely, one must witness that symptom while the baby is eating that particular food, witness the symptom abate when the food is eliminated from the child's diet, and witness it resume when the food is once again fed to the baby. This checking system is called "elimination diet with food challenge." The symptoms may include a runny nose, wheezing, vomiting and abdominal pain, diarrhea, mood changes, and skin lesions, particularly hives and eczema—obviously, a lot of symptoms with a lot of possible causes. But we know they are allergic symptoms only if there has been an elimination diet followed by challenge with the suspect food.

Matters are confused even more in the first year of life because a child may display symptoms suggestive of a food allergy on first exposure to the food, have the symptoms abate when the food is stopped, and then tolerate the food very well when it is reintroduced six months (more or less) later.

"So, just because she has a reaction doesn't mean she can never touch that food again."

"That's right."

By avoiding solid-food mixtures, a reaction can be clearly related to a specific food, and that food avoided for a while. If a mixture causes a reaction, there is no way of knowing which food in the mixture to eliminate. It is also a fact that it may take four or five days before a reaction to a new food becomes evident. It is best, therefore, to let about a week pass before introducing a new food. Otherwise, you can't be sure if a reaction is a delayed one from the familiar food or is being caused by the new one.

"After the rice cereal, I wait a while before starting something else. What do I start next?" Mrs. Richardson asked. "Strained food? Junior food? Fruits? Vegetables?"

"I would stay with the strained foods at first—maybe until a year or so, and stick with the small jar if there is a choice. The only difference between strained and junior foods is in the texture and the particle size. The strained foods are smoother and have a smaller particle size than the junior foods. Children tend to adapt to their texture better at the start. It will not be long before you can change over to the junior foods, usually by the time the baby is a year old. As far as their caloric and nutrient content is concerned, they are essentially the same.

"The choice of a vegetable or a fruit next is up to you, but I'd advise vegetables. Some of the older baby books suggest giving fruits as the first solid foods after cereals because they are sweet and, as a result, babies almost always go for them. They do, which is one reason why I think it is better to try vegetables first."

Vegetables First

"We know that babies in the first week of life are able to discriminate between sugar water and plain water. When given the choice, they prefer the sugar water. The implications of this early preference are fascinating, especially if you believe that food preferences and habits are established early in infancy. We used to think that babies had no ability to discriminate among foods on the basis of taste—that texture was all they reacted to—so that it made no difference what foods were offered. Since this is not the case, and if they are actually able to establish preferences on the basis of taste, then maybe we should be more concerned about adding too much sugar, *or* salt, to their diets early on.

"Strained and junior fruits contain almost twice as many calories as their vegetable counterparts because of the increased amount of carbohydrate in the fruits. Sugars and salt are no longer added to commercial baby foods, but the inherent sweetness of fruits is still there."

"So, by starting vegetables first," Mrs. Richardson said, "I might make it less likely that Elizabeth will have a 'sweet tooth' later on."

"Yes. And you might make it more likely that she will grow up enjoying her vegetables."

"Do you have any proof that starting with vegetables has this effect?" she asked.

"No. Not yet. But the speculation seems reasonable. I have heard of a family with two growing boys. One showed a distinct preference for apple juice. As an infant, he had been started on fruits before receiving vegetables. The other loved grapefruit juice. He had started on vegetables first. And there have been other anecdotal reports along these lines. But the scientific proof is yet to come. I can tell you with assurance, however, that there is no harm in giving vegetables first."

"The same procedure as before?"

"The same. One at a time—not mixed with anything else. Get the plain, not the creamed vegetables. A week between everything new, and if Elizabeth doesn't like it at first, don't force her. Wait a day and try again."

"Does it matter which vegetable I start with?"

"Not really, except that babies have strong preferences for colors. They are more likely to put something bright, like carrots, into their mouths. However, there are a lot of other vegetables to choose from. Leave the ones with stronger tastes, like onions or cabbage, for later on. Again, avoid the creamed vegetables at first—they provide more calories, an added renal solute load, and an increased chance of allergic reaction."

As I went on to explain to Mrs. Richardson, parents should

be sure to read the labels on the strained and junior food preparations, since many of them are prepared with orange juice and other additives, making the chance of a difficult-to-diagnose reaction more likely. There is little difference calorically or nutritionally between the starchy fruit preparations and the so-called desserts. Both are relatively high in calories compared to vegetables and contain a lot of carbohydrates. Fruit juices are lower in calories than fruits alone, yet higher in vitamin C content than the fruit preparations.

I recommend apple juice as a better juice to start with than orange juice, since I've heard of fewer reactions to it. Also, normal development plays a role in the introduction of fruit juices. They are best started when the baby is old enough to drink from a cup, somewhere around nine to eleven months. You should not add fruit juices to a bottle to be given to a baby at bedtime. The increased carbohydrate content of this mixture can contribute significantly to the development of dental cavities.

Apple juice and orange juice are the only baby-food juices made with single fruits; the other juices are mixtures of more than one fruit juice. All of the strained or junior juice preparations—orange, apple, or the mixtures—have more sugar and calories than freshly squeezed juice or the canned fruit juices adults drink.

Egg yolks—not the whites—are also suitable for the solid-food beginner. Egg yolk contains iron, fats, and vitamin D.

"The reason for separating the yolk from the white," I went on to explain to Mrs. Richardson, "is . . ."

"Allergies!" said Mrs. Richardson.

"That's right. The white contains as many complex proteins as meats and should be saved for the mature digestive system of the slightly older child."

"So I should put off giving her meats. Until what age?" she asked.

"There is no age. It used to be thought that meats and high proteins were not to be started until after a year, then it was nine months, now it is any time after six months. I'm still conservative on this score and tend to advise waiting until nine months for meats, egg whites and other complex proteins. I would certainly save them for last—after the cereals, vegetables, and fruits."

"I see foods labeled 'high-meat dinners,' 'soups,' and 'dinners.' What does all this mean?"

"Where the meat appears first in the variety name of the dinner, like 'turkey with vegetables,' it means that the meat is the chief ingredient. In a high-meat dinner, there is less protein than in meat dinners alone, but more protein than in the soups, in which meat is just another ingredient along with vegetables. Meat dinners are prepared with a lower fat content than found in homemade meat meals. They are a good source, but a relatively expensive one, of iron and the B vitamins."

"Now that I understand what all of these things are, there's another question. Why should I use them at all? What if I want to prepare foods for Elizabeth myself?"

"Go right ahead. You don't have to use any of the commercial foods. Home preparation takes a bit longer, so it is not as convenient. In all other respects, however, it's an excellent way to feed your child. Just be careful of one or two things," I said, and proceeded to explain further.

Home-Prepared Foods

The reasons for *starting* solid foods are to provide iron and to enable the child to accept new foods easily. The cereal preparations made for smaller babies are iron fortified. The cereal you would provide at home is not. So either find other sources of iron for your baby, such as egg yolks and, later on, meats, or use the iron-fortified baby cereals. Since the commercially prepared foods contain a good deal of water, the amount of iron contained in them is less than that in an equivalent amount of the same food prepared at home. Also be aware of the fact that so-called animal iron—e.g., iron derived from animal

sources like meats, fish, poultry, and egg yolks—is more readily absorbed by the child than is vegetable iron, e.g., spinach.
Cow's milk does not have enough iron. As the volume of cow's
milk increases, egg yolk, meats, and iron-containing vegetables
must also increase in the diet. Use the baby-food dry cereals,
diluted with water, if there is any question that the baby will be
getting enough iron.

Since home preparations of vegetables and fruits have less
water content than those commercially prepared, they have
more calories per teaspoon and a higher renal solute load. I
still recommend home-prepared foods whenever possible, because, except possibly in the case of iron, the parent knows
what the baby is getting. I do, however, think the following
suggestion is very important: prepare the baby's portion of
food before seasoning the remainder to the family's taste.

Until 1977, commercially prepared baby foods often had more
salt than home-prepared foods. Salt was added to make them
tastier—to the parent. The child does not need the salt and is
relatively unaffected by the bland taste of unsalted food. Recognition of this fact and cautioning by child nutritionists about
the possible ill effects of high-salt diets, including high blood
pressure later in life, led to the removal of salt by the baby-
food producers in the late 1970s. Recently, investigators looked
at the relative salt content of commercial and home-prepared
foods and found that home-prepared foods frequently had *more*
salt, largely because mother or father, whoever did the cooking, seasoned the food to his or her own tastes.

The same may be said for sugars. Many of the commercially
prepared foods have a low fat content. This means that more
of the calories provided in the food will be in the form of carbohydrates, such as sucrose, lactose, dextrose, and corn and
tapioca starches. The starches are primarily for texture and may
not be absorbed well by the infant, who doesn't have enough
of the enzyme required for their digestion. Even though
homemade foods have more calories, they have a better balance of proteins, carbohydrates, and fats. The sweetness that

comes from high carbohydrates in some food is not only unnecessary, but also, as mentioned before, might predispose the
baby to a preference for sweets later on in life. Fortunately,
some commercial baby-food manufacturers have also removed
excessive sugar from their product. Read the label—it has the
answers.

Because of the higher renal solute load of home-prepared
foods, the baby should also be given water, at least a bottle or
two a day, or breast milk.

"How do I coordinate the feeding of breast milk with the
feeding of solids?" asked Mrs. Richardson.

"At the beginning, when breast milk still provides the substantial part of Elizabeth's diet, let her empty one breast first,
in order to keep your milk supply stimulated. Then offer her
some cereal or vegetables. See what she takes, and then offer
the other breast. As she becomes more and more interested in
the solid foods, you can offer her less and less from the breast.
This will lead to a decrease in milk supply as the demand drops
off. The transition should come somewhere around nine
months—a good age to wean Elizabeth from the breast (although some pediatricians feel that if mother *and* baby are satisfied breast-feeding should continue longer). It is very
important, however, that milk still be a significant part of the
diet. But foods with high protein are also important for the
baby. The protein content of vegetables, fruits, and rice cereal
is low. Egg whites, meats, chicken, fish, high-protein cereal—
all the foods we said we'd put off until later—are excellent
sources of protein. Until they are taken in good quantity, milk
remains the major source of protein."

"I think I understand," she said. "Can you just write out
your recommendations?"

"I'd be glad to. But don't follow them too religiously. Experiment with what she likes. Look at it this way: you can do no
harm. As far as the order of events goes, start with cereals,
then vegetables, then fruits and some egg yolks. Wait until

somewhere around nine months and then introduce the meats and other high-protein foods. These are just guidelines. Let Elizabeth have some say in the process. It is, after all, a two-way interaction: your offering and her accepting. Without her accepting, there's no interaction. Without interaction, it's like force-feeding."

From Bottle-Feeding to Solids

If Mrs. Richardson had been bottle-feeding her baby for the past six months, the philosophy would be the same. There is merit to the argument that babies who are drinking breast milk, with its higher carbohydrate content than cow's milk, need high-protein foods to balance their diet, whereas children on high-protein cow's milk need more carbohydrates. The child maintained on infant formula from six months to a year has needs not unlike those of the child on human breast milk. Although the protein content of formula is still slightly higher than that of breast milk, it is not as high as in cow's milk that has not been modified. The recommendation of the American Academy of Pediatrics is that children weaned from the breast should be fed formula until a year of age.

The procedures for introducing solid foods to the bottle-fed baby are no different, either. At the onset, the baby can be offered milk, then some solid foods, and then more milk. Cereals and fruit juices do not belong in a bottle.

"Is it true that babies who are fed formula tend to be more obese in later life than babies brought up on breast milk?" asked Mrs. Richardson.

"The answer to that is not yet clear. There has been recent research in England that shows no difference between the two groups. However, there does seem to be a temptation to 'finish the bottle,' and that might lead to overfeeding. There is also a tendency among parents who bottle-feed to add solid foods to the diet earlier. Solids, with their higher caloric and carbohydrate content, might predispose to overfeeding also.

But it is definitely going to take more research to figure out the connection, if any, between these two forms of infant feeding and later obesity."

Tooth Development and Fluoride

"You mentioned that carbohydrates in the bottle may lead to cavities. You also said I should mix my baby's cereal with water, particularly if it is fluoridated, to protect the teeth. Elizabeth's six months old now. When should I expect her to have teeth, and since she doesn't have any yet, why on earth am I worried about fluoride?"

"Although you weren't able to see it," I responded, "Elizabeth's primary teeth began to calcify during your pregnancy. The areas of the teeth where cavities usually form calcified after birth. Some of her teeth had completed their enamel formation when she was as young as a month and a half to two months of age. Since three or four months of age, many of her permanent teeth have been hardening. All of this has happened under her gums, where you couldn't see it going on.

"We know that if fluoride is incorporated into the outer layers of enamel, the baby's teeth will be more resistant to cavity formation. Since enamel is completely formed in some of the primary teeth by one and a half months of age, addition of fluoride to the diet in the first month is theoretically useful. Fluoride is absorbed from the digestive system and able to reach the new teeth through the blood. And, although the quantity is not great, it is likely that some fluoride reaches the baby in the breast milk.

"We know for certain that the secondary or permanent teeth are undergoing active enamel formation from four months of age until sixteen years of age, when the third and last molar is finally enamelled. By making sure that fluoride, usually in the form of fluoridated water, is added to the baby's diet, we decrease considerably the child's susceptibility to cavities later in life."

"And if you don't live in an area where the water is fluoridated?" asked Mrs. Richardson.

"Most dentists recommend fluoride drops added to the diet after the child is six months old."

"Why not from birth?"

"Because the chance of overdoing the drops is greater than if fluoride is added to the baby's water. Fluoride-overdose symptoms can show up in a 'mild' form as a pitting in the formation of enamel. In the severe form, after a sudden fluoride overdose, there can be nausea, vomiting and abdominal pain, and maybe even convulsions. Given these possible toxic effects, it is safer to start at six months when the amount required versus the amount causing toxicity is not so close. Fluoride will still have a positive effect when started at that age."

"When can I expect to see her teeth erupt?" was Mrs. Richardson's next question.

"The variability is considerable," I explained. "On the average, six to seven months for the lower central incisor. But it may come earlier. I've seen some cases in which teeth are already erupted at birth, but that's extreme. Or eruption might come later. Some babies have no teeth at fourteen months. If the date of first eruption goes beyond this, we can X-ray her jaw to see if her teeth are there. They are absent *very* rarely. Although her primary teeth are very important in guaranteeing good placement and jaw formation for her permanent teeth, they are certainly not necessary for nutrition in the first year. And if they erupt too soon, they can sometimes make breast-feeding more painful."

Weaning to the Cup

"That brings up one last, very important concern," said Mrs. Richardson. "When, how, and onto what do I wean her?"

Mrs. Richardson's concern raises what many consider to be the last major issue for the breast-feeding mother in the first year. However, it must be pointed out that calling it the final issue is somewhat arbitrary. Mothers, after all, may wean their children from the breast at any age, from one week (or earlier) to one year (or later). In some cultures, two- and three-year-old children are still being breast-fed because breast milk may represent the best source of protein in that culture's ecology.

Although it may seem obvious that the decision to wean should be left solely to the mother, there are many instances when this is not so. Relatives and friends may exert a lot of pressure in either direction. Mothers may respond to a guilt-laden challenge such as "You're not going to stop *now* are you? Just when things were going so well?" by continuing even when they would rather not. It won't take long for the joy to evaporate from that feeding situation. Or, conversely, a mother may feel compelled to stop by the social sanction implied by questions such as "Aren't you going too far with that? I mean, really, don't you think you've made your point?" These are usually the comments of persons feeling less than comfortable in their own roles as parents.

The fact is, many mothers are going on to breast-feed beyond the first two months. A recent study reviewing breast-feeding trends from 1971 to 1979 showed that the percentage of mothers breast-feeding their babies at five to six months (including those using supplemental formulas) had risen from 5.5 percent in 1971 to 23 percent in 1979. Many mothers feel that once they make it through the difficulties of the first two months, they are ready to go on for an indefinite period.

"So when should I stop breast-feeding?" pondered Mrs. Richardson. "Is there some time that you consider better than others?"

I went on to discuss my opinions and preferences, and the rationale behind them.

Ideally, the baby should be on breast milk for the first five to six months for all of the nutritional, immunological, and anti-allergic reasons already noted. Weaning between five months and one year is probably most desirable. Beyond one year, the process may become more difficult. Older children, as a rule, are not as adaptable to the change as younger children. Also, waiting until after the first birthday may mean delaying the use of a cup. Babies accustomed to the breast for so long may find a cup entertaining but may not readily accept it as an implement of nutrition.

I recommend weaning between six months and a year, and by this I mean stopping breast-feeding altogether during those months. Partial weaning or the addition of a supplementary bottle can be instigated earlier, but at least not until after two months, when the stability and sufficiency of the mother's breast milk supply is assured. The most immediate need for a supplementary bottle is when the breast milk supply is insufficient. Although uncommon, this case is more likely to occur after four months, when the baby's rapid growth and increased appetite may outstrip the mother's supplies. (Adequacy of breast milk nourishment can be determined by plotting the baby's growth along the appropriate curves of the length and weight charts in Appendix 1.)

Whether for need or convenience, the supplementary bottle started at five to six months represents the first step toward weaning, since, used as a substitute for one feeding, it leads to a decrease in stimulation of milk production. However, many mothers who have been breast-feeding successfully are reluctant to start the baby on a bottle at all. They prefer weaning from the breast right to a cup. This makes sense in many ways. There is no need to make an investment in nursing bottles, nipples, and formula. The baby has to undergo only one weaning—breast to cup—instead of two—breast to bottle and bottle to cup. And there is no chance this way that the bottle will become a bedtime pacifier.

For successful one-step weaning, the baby should be kept on the breast until nine months or so. Trying to make a sudden transition, however, is unlikely to be successful; offering expressed breast milk or formula in a cup at around seven months helps ease the conversion. As the amount of cup milk (human or formula) becomes greater, the amount of milk supplied directly from the breast can be allowed to diminish. This way, by the time the baby is ten to eleven months old, most of the infant's milk intake can be from a cup. The infant may still be suckling at the breast for his own and his mother's psychological needs, but once it becomes evident that enough nourishment can be supplied through solid foods and milk from a cup, it will become easier for both to relinquish the attachment.

Weaning from the bottle to a cup is in many respects the same. Formula will suffice until the baby is a year old. The same timing of the gradual shift from bottle to cup, starting at six months and leading to weaning before a year, should be successful.

"I heard of a friend," said Mrs. Richardson, "who didn't bother with a gradual transition at all. Just one day, bang! the bottle wasn't there. Oh, sure, the baby had been drinking juice from a cup, but I'm sure she never thought that milk came from a cup."

"And what happened?" I asked.

"There was some disagreement between the mother and the baby for a couple of days, and not much milk got in. But she made up for it by offering more juice and more solid foods. It worked."

"I guess so," I said. "I've heard of that working when the child was over a year old and the bottle had become somewhat superfluous to the rest of the diet. How old was she?"

"About a year," she said.

"We have to remember that every child is different. Don't be afraid to experiment, but do try and avoid 'confrontational nutrition.' There's no point setting up a conflict when there doesn't have to be one," I said. "That type of abrupt, cold-turkey weaning is more difficult for the breast-feeding mother. She will go on making milk and may become engorged if she stops too early. But it can be done."

"How much milk per day should the baby be drinking by a year of age?" asked Mrs. Richardson.

"Estimates vary," I said. "Assume a quart to a quart and a half. That way, at least half of Elizabeth's calories will come from milk—and by a year of age, it can certainly be cow's milk."

"Skim milk?" she asked.

"Only after the first birthday," I answered. "Before that, babies need the essential fatty acids which are skimmed off skim milk. The milk fats are the major source of fat in their diet at that age. If you cut down on their amount, the calories will still come from somewhere—either from carbohydrates (increasing the risk of dental cavities and obesity) or from protein (increasing the renal solute load and the risk of allergies). However, skim milk can be used, wisely, after a year.

Weaning the child at the end of the first year constitutes a true landmark in the baby's nutritional development. It is also a psychological and social landmark. The child has, in a literal as well as a symbolic way, made the first step toward independence. The child is now free from the breast. Mother and father remain in their roles of ultimate caretakers, providing whatever food the child wants to eat. But just as the requirements for milk begin to diminish, so does the child's complete dependency on the parents. Total independence is a long way off, but the beginning of the second year of life leaves no question that that day is inevitably (and to some parents, a bit sadly) going to come.

CHAPTER 7

Feeding Your Child: From the First Year to School Time

Nutrition and Neurological Development

Although the title of this chapter is expressed in chronological terms, the first year to school time, the nutritional behavior covered is related more to the developmental age of the child than to the child's age in years or months. Chronological age can serve only as a rough indicator of what a child is developmentally capable of doing, since all children do not mature at the same rate.

It is not surprising that nutritional growth very closely parallels neurodevelopmental growth. Throughout the animal kingdom, developmental growth is accompanied by growth in capability for self-sustenance, since the taking in of nourishment is necessary for survival. In this respect, *Homo sapiens* is no different from other species. We go through a sequence of developmental stages which determines the sequence of our nutritional progress. The developmental sequence begins with the control of the head and neck, and then control of the trunk.

[*90*]

The development of truncal control is the beginning of what we call "balance." Balance is essential. Without it, our hands would have to be used for support and would not be free for gathering and feeding.

In human beings, the feeding process of the infant is well adapted to developmental capability. The poor head control and total lack of hand control of the newborn necessitated feeding at a nipple. Other developmental reflexes support this process: for example, the extrusor reflex, which gets milk from the nipple, and the rooting reflex, which helps the infant find the nipple. These feeding reflexes continue until four months at least, at which time the extrusor reflex disappears and the child's head and neck control improves. Balance, however, is still poor, a reflection of poor trunk control. The five-month-old baby not only has good head control but is also developing the truncal control that will allow sitting without support when the baby is six months old. Balance at five months is good enough so that hands can be used to bring food to the mouth, but not so good as to allow moving around to gather things out of immediate reach. That may not happen until the infant is eight to nine months old, when crawling and creeping begin. But walking, at a year old, is the ultimate demonstration of body balance, allowing mobility *and* freedom of hand use.

Before this event occurs, however, the baby goes through a developmental progression of use of the hands, similar to the progression of use of head and trunk. At birth, the hands remain at either side of the body, out of the infant's range of vision. The hands are obviously of no immediate use to the child if the child cannot see them. They gradually move into an area where they become visible. By about three months, the baby's hands have moved to the midline of the child's sight. By three and a half to four months the baby is actually capable of reaching for a close-by object and grasping it.

Once the infant is older, the grasp will be a neat finger-and-thumb pincer grasp, useful for picking up small objects, but at four months all the baby can muster is a clumsy clutch of a large block between the outside of the palm and the fourth and fifth finger. This clutching looks more like an accident than a deliberate grasp.

When five months old, the infant not only reaches and grasps a block or similar object (which is now held in the middle of the palm), but tries to put it into the mouth—a first step toward self-feeding. Children at this age, however, do not put things in their mouths to swallow them. They do so for the oral gratification of feeling them on their gums. A month or so later, when given a biscuit a baby will move it around the gums until it finally gets so soft from mouthing that some of it will be swallowed. This is the age at which teething biscuits are a good idea. They are purposely made to flake easily so that whatever portion of them gets past the front of the mouth won't obstruct the baby's windpipe and cause choking.

Small food objects, such as peanuts and raisins, are not a good thing to have within reach of the baby at this age. This is the age a baby starts picking such objects up. By seven months the infant is able to grasp them with some part of the index finger and thumb. However, the entire action is still rather awkward. Because the raisin or peanut may be held at the base of the finger, where it is trapped by the thumb, it is difficult to get it into the mouth. Nevertheless, keep such objects away from infants. They will try eating them until they succeed and could end up choking themselves if the object blocks breathing. It is a good age, though, to give the infant larger finger foods to play with and put into the mouth. Let infants at this age feed themselves a biscuit or a diced piece of carrot. They'll enjoy it more if they are allowed to put it in their own mouths.

The development of skilled use of the hands culminates, to some extent, at ten to eleven months with the discrete thumb-finger grasp. Like a tiny pair of calipers, the finger and thumb reach out, and come down on the target from above. The infant picks up whatever catches her attention, brings it closer to her face to examine it and—pop—into her mouth. Now, nutritionally, the baby is really in business. Not only does the food go into her mouth, but the baby is now ready to chew on it and swallow it. At this point, you'd have to say that the infant is ready for anything—whether lumpy junior foods or food from the table cut up so that it can be managed.

"So," said Mrs. Richardson, "let me see how all this information about development compares with Elizabeth's progress." She had brought her baby book with her to show me on Elizabeth's first birthday. She turned its pages of pictures and other memorabilia and started reminiscing. . . .

"She liked her teething biscuit at six months. You're right, look! Everything was going into her mouth anyway," she said, pointing at a photograph. "And she must have been developing—well I guess they were already developed—she must have been pushing her first teeth through, which is why she liked it so much. She had two teeth by the next month." She went back to her perusal of the book. "It's interesting," she observed; "teeth started coming out right around the time when she began to chew things instead of just mouth them.

"At seven months she was eating—at least playing with finger foods—because she could use her fingers. Look." She pointed to a picture of her daughter with a lot of food around her mouth, on her bib, and pretty much all over the tray in front of her. "It used to drive my husband crazy," she smiled. "He couldn't stand having *his* daughter such a mess. But he got over it. We both realized it was better letting her feed herself a little."

"She seems to be having a great time," I observed.

"Oh, she loved it. Here she is at ten months. Do you see how she's holding that piece of biscuit?" She pointed to the picture. "Right between the thumb and forefinger, just like you said she should. That wasn't so long ago, either." She glanced up at me a bit hesitantly. "You know, we were both worried that you'd be angry with us for having given her table foods."

"Me, angry at you for that?" I was surprised. "Why?"

"Oh, because you had said she probably wouldn't be ready for table foods until her first birthday."

"Did I really sound that dogmatic? I certainly didn't mean to. Each child develops differently, at a slightly different rate. Those of us, parents and pediatricians, who take care of kids have to be sensitive to each child's developmental peculiarities and tailor our expectations and demands to fit them. If Elizabeth was ready to eat table foods and able to tolerate them before a year, even before ten months, that's fine. All I meant to imply by what I said earlier was that table foods wouldn't be a large part of her diet until she was a year old."

"She still drinks a lot of milk."

"How much? Three to four bottles?" She nodded. "And the rest is junior food?"

"Actually, we've switched pretty much over to the food everyone else is eating at home," said Mrs. Richardson.

This is typical of how a major transition is normally made that changes the whole nature of a child's nutrition. The child at one year of life (or thereabouts) no longer needs to eat a special formula prepared by a pharmaceutical company or a special baby food made by a baby-food producer. Beyond the first year, the child is developmentally and nutritionally in a position to eat what the rest of the family is eating. Her neurodevelopment is accompanied by maturation of her kidney function, which helps her cope with the higher renal solute load of table food, and by the maturation of the digestive system, which makes it less likely that a child will develop allergic reactions to the more complex proteins of the family food. As she grows, the diet becomes less and less special and more and more like everyone else's.

Assessing Adequate Nutrition

When Mrs. Richardson brought in Elizabeth on her first birthday, she did not ask if her child was taking enough, as she had on earlier visits. Instead it was: "What's her height and weight on your scales?" And when her little girl had been weighed and measured, she plotted both measurements on her home growth chart, which she had brought along. She then looked up with some satisfaction.

"Three times her birth weight." She smiled happily. "And still between the 25th and 50th percentile for both height and weight." Then she frowned slightly. "I know she's growing fine," Mrs. Richardson said. "And I also know that the breast milk, the formula, and the strained and junior foods are designed and fortified to make sure she eats a balanced diet. But now she's getting away from all of those. She's beginning to eat what the rest of us are eating. How do I know she's getting enough of everything? How do I plan her diet now?"

"The increase of height and weight along the appropriate growth curve is still an excellent indicator of balanced nutrition," I said, "as is her normal developmental examination. You don't grow well if you are malnourished, even if only one part of the balanced diet is missing. Take, for instance, children with selective protein malnutrition. The condition is called 'kwashiorkor.' The kids may look fat because of the carbohydrates they are eating. In fact, they are sometimes referred to as 'sugar babies.' And they actually continue to gain weight along their proper weight curve. But their ability to gain in height without the protein necessary for new cell formation is severely impeded. As a result, their weight-to-height ratio becomes distinctly abnormal. Now, I'll grant you that kwashiorkor is very rarely seen in this country, but the point is that small deficits, even isolated deficits in amino acids or essential fatty acids, show up as abnormalities in growth and development."

"What you're saying is that if Elizabeth is growing 'normally' I don't have to worry. But it also sounds as if things would have to go a long way to the bad side before I'd be able to tell," said Mrs. Richardson. "Tell me how to plan a diet for the baby so that I don't have to worry."

The choice of diet for the one-year-old is not significantly different from that for other preschool members of the family. One thing that must be remembered, however, is that for the coming year and the year after, things may not be as regular for the one-year-old as they were before. A balanced diet now becomes balanced more on a per-week basis than on a per-day or per-meal basis. The driving stimulus for appetite over the first year was the child's rapid growth rate, a rate that caused the child's birth weight to triple by the first birthday. Growth slows in the second year. The child who went from 7 pounds at birth to 21 or 22 pounds at one year may normally gain only another 5 or 6 pounds from the first birthday to the second. The child who gained 10 inches in the first year may creep up only another 5 over the following year. Appetite and calorie needs diminish accordingly. Babies require 120 kilocalories per kilogram of body weight, that is, 55 calories per pound, during the early months of life. By the time they are one year old, because of the slowing up in growth velocity, the requirement is 95 to 100 kilocalories per kilogram (45 calories per pound). This means the 7.5-pound newborn who needed 420 calories a day in the first month grew up to be the 17-pound six-month-old who needed 930 calories a day—a sizable leap of more than twice the number of calories needed each day. This same child becomes the 21- to 22-pound one-year-old who needs 1,000 calories each day. Now the increase is only 70 calories, which amounts to an added caloric requirement for the one-year-old that could be satisfied with an extra 3.5 ounces of milk.

"So I shouldn't expect my baby to eat too much at meals," interpreted Mrs. Richardson accurately.

"Not only that," I said, "but an overexpectation of what the baby should be taking can lead to an awful lot of battles. Remember what we said about feeding your baby in the first six months: trust her instincts. She'll eat when she's hungry. Just be sure that when she does want to eat, you offer her the right choices."

"How do I know what's right?" was Mrs. Richardson's next question.

The Recommended Dietary Allowances

Every five years or so, the National Academy of Science publishes *The Recommended Dietary Allowances* (RDA), intended "to provide standards serving as a goal for good nutrition." It was anticipated with the first publication of the dietary allowances in 1943, and it has proved to be true, that the recommendations would change with time as our knowledge of what constituted "good nutrition" expanded.

The *Recommended Dietary Allowances* gave seed to the United States *Recommended Daily Allowances* (US RDA), which tells us what is required for good nutrition on a *daily* basis. The percentage of the recommended daily allowance of particular nutrients provided in packaged foods is often listed on the manufacturer's package, can, or bottle.

The problem with using Recommended Dietary Allowances or US Recommended Daily Allowances is that they are recommendations for populations—large groups of people—not for individuals. The needs of individual members of the whole population for a particular nutrient are highly variable. Some will need more than the average person, some will need less than the average. The RDA's are not intended merely to meet the needs of the average person, since that would mean underestimating the needs of some members of the group. As stated in the 1980 edition, estimation of the recommended allowances follows essentially four steps: "(1) Estimating the average requirement of a population for a given nutrient and the variability of requirement within that population. (2) Increasing the average requirement by an amount sufficient to meet the needs of nearly all members of that population. (3) Increasing the allowance to account for inefficient utilization by the body of the nutrients as consumed (poor absorption, poor conversion of precursor to active form, etc.). (4) Using judgment in interpreting and extrapolating allowances when information on requirement is limited."

In order to estimate the average requirement infants have

for a given nutrient, for example, normally growing breast-fed babies were studied for the amount of the nutrient they ingested in breast milk. Since nutrients in breast milk are almost totally absorbed, the amount ingested was used to define the requirements of that nutrient for normal growth. With some nutrients, dietary requirements were determined on the evidence of deficiencies (rashes, failure to thrive, etc.) when the nutrient was either inadvertently left out of the solution given to infants on total intravenous feeding, or provided in too small an amount.

The allowances, as noted above, take into account the inefficient utilization of consumed nutrients. Inefficient utilization of iron in infant formulas is a good example of this problem. Iron is more readily absorbed from human milk than from formula. If just the amount of iron found in human milk is added to infant formula, an iron-deficiency state rapidly ensues. In order to compensate for this poor absorption, more iron is recommended for ingestion in the diet. On some packaged foods, the amount of iron is given as "available iron," meaning that the manufacturer has taken the responsibility for estimating how much of the iron provided will actually be absorbed and thus available to satisfy the daily need. "Availability" of other nutrients may also be noted on some packaged foods. These estimates, however, are highly unreliable for specific individuals.

It is evident that the recommended dietary allowances for particular nutrients are overestimates of what many of us need. This is one factor which limits their usefulness for the individual. They are also presented in a form that is useful to the nutritionist and doctor but not particularly to the lay person— milligrams per kilogram, for example, or milligrams per day. There is no translation into everyday food units—ounces of milk, pieces of bread, number of oranges, and the like. This lack is compensated for somewhat by the manufacturers of packaged foods who place nutritional information on the package. They take the *US Recommended Daily Allowances* and tell the consumer what percentage of the recommended allowance is provided in one serving of their product. The *US RDA's* are, however, overestimations, as are the *Recommended Dietary Allowances*. The daily allowances are not to be followed religiously. It can be assumed that failing to achieve 100 percent of a recommended daily allowance one day will be made up in subsequent days if the individual is eating a varied diet. And for the average well-nourished individual, the body will have sufficient stores of a particular nutrient to carry it over a number of days. Consequently, the dietary allowances are best averaged over a five- to eight-day period. At this point, however, the importance of a varied diet must be emphasized. Balance is achieved through variety. Eating the same food type day after day may do no harm—until the body's normal stores of the nutrients not provided by that food type are exhausted. Although such exhaustion may take weeks or months, depending on how restricted the diet is, the end result is diminished health.

The only element of the diet not overestimated by the *Recommended Dietary Allowances* is energy or *calories*. Calories are recommended on the basis of what is needed by the average individual. The National Academy of Science recognizes that the consumption of calories in this country is almost universally a problem of too many rather than not enough.

"This is all very interesting," said Mrs. Richardson, "and I'm glad to know about the *Recommended Dietary Allowances*. I'm also glad to know that I don't have to be obsessed with reading package covers every day and calculating the percentage of daily allowances Elizabeth is eating. But you're not suggesting I do this even on a weekly basis, are you? Even when she gets older?"

"No. Not at all. In fact, as far as I'm concerned you can ignore that information expressed as percentages of daily requirements. Of course, what those numbers are good for is telling you in relative terms what nutrients the product contains after it has been processed, fortified, and so on. For instance, a product that offers you 45 percent of the US RDA for iron, 25 percent of the US RDA for zinc, and less than 2 percent of the US RDA for vitamin C is obviously not a good daily source of vitamin C. It is a moderately good source of zinc, which, in fact, can easily be supplemented in the course of a normal day's diet, and is also a reasonably good source of iron. The point is, you or your child could not go on an extended diet of this product alone without developing severe deficiencies, first of all in vitamin C. But if you balanced your diet by eating fruits for vitamin C and meats or fish for iron and zinc, you would do just fine."

"But, you see," she complained, "you know that fish has a lot of zinc and iron, but how am I supposed to know that? And what do I do about thiamine, riboflavin, and niacin? These always seem to be listed on the outside of the food packages. And it always seems that the food provides only 25 percent of the US RDA."

"Thiamine is vitamin B_1 and is available from many food sources—liver, meat, milk, whole grains, but not polished rice, and from peas, beans, and so on. Riboflavin is available in meat, milk, eggs, green vegetables, and whole grains. Niacin is found mainly in meat and fish, but also in whole grains and green vegetables."

"I'll have to take you shopping with me," she said.

"No. You don't have to take me or any other so-called expert shopping with you. Nor do you have to memorize vitamins available in individual foods or spend your hours in the kitchen with a list of US RDA's in one hand and a calculator in the other. Granted, vitamin content and recommended allowances are helpful to know about. But no one has to get bogged down in their precise measurements," I said. "Look at the food types that provide the three vitamins you just asked about: they are simply meats and fish, whole grains and vegetables, and milk and eggs. Add fruits to this group and you have what nutritionists and dieticians refer to as the Basic Four. The Basic Four can be sort of the busy person's recommended daily allowance. By serving foods from each of these groups, you can just about guarantee that Elizabeth will receive a balanced intake of nutrients."

"You mean, serve one food from each group daily?" asked Mrs. Richardson. "Or at each meal?"

The "Basic Four" and the "Basic Five"

"Either would be fine," I said. "But don't overstuff her with too many calories in the attempt. I think you should use the concept of the Basic Four as you would the RDA's, averaging food types over a five-day period by providing a varied diet. I like the Basic Four idea because it offers an easily remembered way to balance a diet. But I would modify it a bit by making the list less of a Basic Four and more a Basic *Five*. I would make whole grains and vegetables two separate items instead of one."

The reason for the change is that grains and vegetables provide different kinds of proteins. Both are needed for a well-balanced diet. For instance, a family fed only rice but no vegetables would soon develop protein deficiency, whereas a family fed rice and a vegetable would not. Combining grains and vegetables in a single unit as is done in the Basic Four may tend to make people forget that *both* are needed for a balanced diet, particularly if the diet is low in other protein sources, like meat, chicken, or fish.

"So what I'm mainly going to do," summarized Mrs. Richardson, "is provide her with a varied diet—'varied' being the key word—on a daily or weekly basis. If I do that, she'll receive the nutrients she requires for normal growth and development."

"That's right. You'll provide her with essentially the same diet you are feeding the rest of the family," I said.

I then went on to explain that there is another way to look at nutritional planning. Essentially, what we eat is designed to provide us with the energy necessary for survival. Survival means getting along from day to day. The energy provided by our diet keeps our body at the right temperature, keeps our heart and lungs moving, and gives us the power to move around, whether that means running a marathon or lifting a spoon to our mouths. The infant and child, however, have an additional energy requirement. They need energy for growth. This is why the daily energy requirements (energy is expressed in calories) for an average 75-kilogram (165-pound) adult is approximately 25 calories per kilogram, while for a growing 15-kilogram (33-pound) three-year-old, it is 100 calories per kilogram.

Another requirement for growth is protein, not because it is a particularly good energy source, which it is not, but because cell membranes, the nuclei, the DNA and RNA used in duplication of cells, and all the enzymes necessary for cell division and hence growth are made from protein. So it would seem apparent that the growing child has a greater protein requirement than the already grown adult. Memorizing the amount of this protein requirement is unimportant. Recognizing that protein is necessary for growth and that growth velocity decreases after six months of life, leading to a gradual decrease in protein requirements with age, is important.

"What are the foods that provide the most protein?" Mrs. Richardson interrupted.

"Meat, fish, poultry, milk, and eggs," I said.

"But I thought you said that protein was a poor source of energy. Aren't those the foods we are told to eat because they'll give us energy to last us all day?"

"Actually, our parents told us to eat them so we would grow up big and strong. And they were right. Protein equals cell division equals growth. The *energy* in meat, eggs, and milk, however, comes mainly in the form of fat. These foods are rich in fat, and fat is a highly efficient way to ingest calories and store them in the body."

I then went on to talk more about fats and to explain about fatty acids. A small amount of fat contains a lot of calories. Fats are the storage form of energy in the body—not really to be drawn upon until the immediate sources of energy, the carbohydrates, are all used up. Our body fat is what we live on if we have to go a long time without eating or if the demands for energy over a short period of time are so great that our bodies cannot answer them with the sugars. Whenever we take in more energy than we need (i.e., excess calories in the form of carbohydrates, fats, or protein) it is stored as fat in the body. Why, then, do we have to eat any fat at all? Because fat is necessary for the transport across the bowel wall of certain fat-soluble vitamins—vitamins A, D, E, and K. And it is necessary as a source of the primary essential fatty acid, linoleic acid. Essential fatty acids are those fatty acids necessary for normal body function and which the body cannot manufacture for itself.

Linoleic acid is, and serves as the precursor of, what are called "polyunsaturated fatty acids." It is now believed that the essential fatty acids are not only important for maintaining the function and structure of cellular membranes and serving as precursors for a physiologically important group of hormone-like substances called prostaglandins, but they may also be important for prevention of coronary artery disease and other disorders related to blood lipids. This is a highly controversial area, still under active investigation. The polyunsaturated (essential) fatty acids are contained abundantly in vegetable oils. Animal fats contain more saturated fatty acids.

"You mean we should be eating nothing but vegetable oils and margarine?" asked Mrs. Richardson.

"No. You need both saturated and unsaturated. The latest recommendation for adults is that fats make up not more than 35 percent of the total calories ingested, of which slightly less than one-third should be polyunsaturated fats. Again, balance the diet."

"And for kids it's the same?" she asked.

"Nearly the same," I said. "If they are over one year of age, fats should constitute somewhere around 40 percent of their total caloric intake, protein approximately 10 to 12 percent, and carbohydrates the rest, roughly 48 percent."

"So is this an age when I can safely begin skim milk?" she asked.

"Yes. But only because I'm counting on Elizabeth's receiving adequate essential fatty acids from the rest of her diet. The problem with giving skim milk at an earlier age is that in the young infant, milk is the *only* source of fats in the diet. Skimming off the fat not only removes those essential fatty acids but also reduces the number of calories and alters considerably the proportion of the calories that come from protein and carbohydrates. Instead of protein being 12 percent and carbohydrates 48 percent, the percentages become closer to fifty-fifty. This increases the renal solute load considerably."

"What's the difference between skim milk and 2 percent milk?"

"Skim milk contains around 0.1 percent fat. Whole milk has 3.25 percent fat. Two percent milk is in between. The value of any low fat milk is only that you can reduce the amount of cholesterol and saturated fatty acids in Elizabeth's diet and substitute for them with vegetable-derived polyunsaturated fatty acids. You still want to keep her on a diet in which 40 percent of her calories come as fats."

"That means 48 percent of her diet should be sugar," she calculated. "Isn't that an awful lot?"

"Don't forget, all carbohydrates are not sugar, or at least not what we ordinarily consider sugar—the white table sugar called sucrose. A lot of carbohydrates are complex starches, the kind you find in potatoes and other starchy foods. They differ from sucrose in their nutritional value because the foods they are a part of also provide necessary vitamins and minerals. Sucrose comes without any such accompanying nutrients, and may also be a cause of dental caries—two reasons to keep it at a minimum."

"Why bother eating it at all?"

"Well, I know of a lot of families who only use it in cooking, and some who don't use it at all. It does have nutritional value as a ready source of energy."

"So instead of table sugar I should be giving Elizabeth carbohydrates in her diet in the form of starchy foods . . ."

"Like potatoes, corn, beans, and grains such as cereals, macaroni, and bread," I interjected. "Notice they are all highly nutritious foods, not even counting the carbohydrates.

"I think it's reasonable to use these starches as important sources of carbohydrates, particularly now that Elizabeth is over a year old. When she was under six months of age she wasn't able to digest starches efficiently. Her ability to do that has increased since then and should be adequate by now."

"And, I guess, also fruits," she added.

"Yes, fruits are an excellent choice of sweets. They provide different kinds of sugar in addition to the sucrose found in candies and most desserts. Fruits also provide the fibrous texture that helps clean the sugar off the teeth."

"Now, what is the story about fiber in her diet? Is it as necessary as everybody says?" Mrs. Richardson asked.

Dietary Fiber

The fiber that Mrs. Richardson is curious about is resistant to digestion by the gastrointestinal tract. It is found in abundance in vegetables, fruits, and grains and is made up of cellulose and other compounds which provide much of the structure of plants. Sometimes the fiber content of foods is referred to as crude fiber and sometimes as dietary fiber. Crude fiber is what is left over after a food has been treated with acids and alkali similar to the substances that aid digestion in the stomach and small intestine. Some of the fiber present in the food is lost in this process. The total amount of fiber in the food before the acid/alkali treatment is called dietary fiber and is obviously greater than the crude fiber.

Fiber provides the bulk or roughage of a diet. It is a diet component that has been gradually disappearing as we purify and process foods more and more. Some researchers believe that the lack of bulk in our diet has contributed to the increased number of certain diseases, the so-called diseases of civilization. These include diverticulosis (a disease of the intestines), cardiovascular disease, cancer of the large intestine, and adult-onset diabetes. The evidence for this association is not conclusive, however.

"What does fiber do?" asked Mrs. Richardson.

"It's not entirely understood," I answered. "Apparently, it has good effects and bad effects. The bad effects are seen particularly if you eat too much of it.

"The good effects of fiber relate to easier bowel movements and the fact that the stool contains more water. We all know that eating more roughage has been used as a preventive for constipation for generations. Our grandparents certainly knew it, which is why we were fed fruits—"an apple a day keeps the doctor away"—and bran cereals—"100% bran flakes: the natural laxative"—as children. In some cases, increased fiber in the diet leads to a reduction in serum cholesterol, possibly by absorbing bile acids and increasing their excretion in the feces. Bile acids, which are necessary for the digestion of fat in the intestines, are made up in part of cholesterol. This may explain why, as the fiber content of the diet increases, tying up more bile acids, less fat is absorbed and more is excreted in the stool.

"The potentially bad effects of a high-fiber diet relate to the effect fiber has on absorption of various nutrients. Nitrogen and many of the mineral elements in the diet, like zinc, for instance, are less efficiently absorbed in a very high-fiber diet."

"Are you saying we should keep fiber out of our diet, then?" asked Mrs. Richardson.

"No. Not at all. The only situations where it could have a seriously ill effect are when the diet is marginally deficient in mineral nutrients such as zinc and nitrogen or when it is unusually high in fiber content."

"How high is high?"

"I can't give you a number because I don't know, and anyway infants seem to be much better at tolerating fiber in their diets than adults. Too much fiber in our diet makes us feel bloated, gassy, and uncomfortable. Look at it this way. Americans in general could afford to eat a lot more fiber without getting into trouble. Increasing the amount of fresh or unprocessed vegetables and fruits in our diets would generally be a very good thing."

Zinc, Copper, Iodine

"Can we get back to zinc?" Mrs. Richardson asked. "My neighbor has been taking zinc pills for ages—at least since her last pregnancy—and she thinks I should, too. And that I should be giving more zinc to Elizabeth. Do I, does she, really need zinc?"

"Zinc has come to the public's attention in the past five years, probably because with improved technology we've gained a greater understanding of its importance in nutrition. It is a trace element, called a 'micronutrient,' and it is apparently involved in so many enzyme reactions in the body that cells can't grow without it. Fortunately for us, it is also very abundant in nature and in a normal diet—another one of those instances where natural supply seems to meet natural demand.

"It is, however, found in greatest abundance in the most expensive parts of our diet, meats and seafood, and also in eggs. It is also found in whole-grain products—whole wheat, rye, oatmeal—but it's not as well absorbed when it's ingested this way—in part, because of the fiber content of those foods. As an estimate, 60 percent of it is absorbed from meats and seafoods and maybe 20 percent from the vegetable forms.

"As you can imagine, people who cannot afford the meats and seafoods and who don't eat particularly well-balanced diets run the risk of being zinc deficient. When the technology was developed to measure zinc in the blood and in the hair, the number of such people was found to be greater than expected. Zinc deficiency is more common in the lower socio-economic classes than in the upper. The upper and middle classes manage to get enough zinc in their normal daily diets, as long as they are not on a purely vegetarian or some other unusual diet.

"If you don't have enough zinc, how long does it take to show up, and what happens?" she asked.

"Zinc is not well stored in the body in a biologically available form. It also moves out of the system rapidly, which means that zinc deficiency will show up rather fast.

"Early signs of zinc deficiency can be seen in the fetus of a zinc-deficient mother, which is probably the reason your neighbor started taking her supplemental zinc during pregnancy."

"Should I have done that, too?" she asked, somewhat alarmed.

"No, you really didn't need it. Although there is an increased zinc requirement during pregnancy, it's made up for by the increased caloric intake of an increased well-balanced diet. You remember we talked about that? And we continued the increase in caloric intake even after birth in order to supply the extra energy needed for lactation. The baby herself got ample zinc in a well-absorbed form from your breast milk. Bottle-fed babies also get enough if they stay on formula until they eat meats. Formulas are fortified with zinc."

"Can you take too much zinc?"

"Definitely. And it can cause a bad case of vomiting and diarrhea. Zinc is a gastrointestinal irritant. It is also known that a gross excess of zinc can interfere with the absorption of copper. But don't worry. You really don't have to add any zinc to your own or to Elizabeth's diet. A balanced diet is certainly an adequate source of this trace mineral."

"You mentioned copper. Is that important, too? This is beginning to sound more like a hardware store than a doctor's office," she said.

"Copper is also important. But in this hardware store you can browse, you don't have to buy. Copper deficiency is found in some premature babies who are born with low copper reserves and who are brought up on cow's milk for 2 or 3 months. It can also be seen in children suffering from uncommon intestinal disorders in which copper is poorly absorbed and in children suffering from severe malnutrition. But the mineral is so common in our diets—the richest resources are nuts, dried vegetables, meat, and eggs—that you never see copper deficiency in normal children on a well-balanced diet.

"Iodine is another micronutrient I might mention while we're discussing them. Iodine is necessary for the construction of the thyroid hormones. Remember the pictures in our grade-school health books of people who lived far away from the ocean and had developed a thyroid goiter from lack of iodine? Recognition of the cause of goiter led to iodine fortification of much of the salt sold in this country, mainly to serve the noncoastal areas of the country. Coastal areas probably have enough iodine in the environment to serve their daily iodine needs. People living near the coast are also more likely to eat fish, which is another rich source of this micronutrient."

"You've certainly provided me with a lot of information. One question, though. Why are they called micronutrients?" Mrs. Richardson asked.

I explained that micronutrients and trace elements are the same thing. They are nutrients which account for less than 0.01 percent of the total body weight. So, although micronutrients are essential for normal growth and health, the body's requirement for them is very small. This is why, unless you have a disease which specifically interferes with their absorption or consume a diet that is so malnourishing as to be lacking in most of the nutrients necessary for growth, you will not become deficient in these elements.

"One last question?" asked Mrs. Richardson. "How do I balance my baby's diet if she doesn't want it balanced the way I do?"

The Development of Eating Habits

"That's an important question," I answered, "and one that raises the issue of the development of eating habits in general. Eating habits are like other aspects of Elizabeth's development in that they change with time. They are unlike the other aspects of development, however, in being more behaviorally than neurologically or genetically determined. Eating habits are developed in response to patterns set within the child's environment. There is still, however, an interrelationship of neurological and genetic development with behavioral development. Eating habits are the product of both." I went on to discuss this with Mrs. Richardson in terms of her own child's development.

In the first six months, Mrs. Richardson's child will eat whatever is presented to her. This is instinctive behavior related to a need to survive. The only variable in the first months is not what Elizabeth will eat but when she will eat it. Her choice of time to eat is her first step toward exercising some control over her environment. If every time she cries she gets fed, she soon learns that crying is a good way to achieve positive results. Her behavior is said to be reinforced by the parent's response, which is attentive, supportive, and nutritive. Her behavior may also represent, in some extreme cases, a manipulation of the parent, who may be responding not to the child's needs but out of love, anxiety, fear, or guilt.

She refines her control technique as she approaches six months. By then she is able to turn her head and push food on the spoon away or reject a bottle of substance she finds undesirable. Now the infant is in a position not only to control the timing of her diet but also to modify its content to a greater or lesser degree, depending on the disposition of the parent. (It was at this stage that I began to talk to Mrs. Richardson about offering food choices to her baby.) It is important for personality development that the child be allowed to exercise some of this newly acquired control. However, the parent should not yield too readily to the child's early attempts at control. Parents must resist the temptation to offer the child only what will readily be taken, which at this age may be milk or an abundance of fruit. There is nothing nutritionally wrong with either food. What may be wrong is the too permissive attitude of the parent providing them. This parental attitude may persist as the child gets older. The milk and fruit of the six-month-old may become the cookies and soda of the two-year-old.

The other extreme is no better. The parent should not insist that the child eat any and whatever food is provided. A battle ensues when the child, who has, of course, the ultimate say in what goes down the esophagus, adamantly refuses the food. If allowed to continue, this mealtime battle behavior may become more of a response to the mealtime situation than to the food.

By offering a choice between two equally nutritious foods, the parent allows the child to exercise the control over environment necessary for normal development, while at the same time guaranteeing good nutrition. If Elizabeth refuses both choices, and milk is still a major part of her diet, Mrs. Richardson should offer her milk, but keep offering the choices as the child gets older. When she reaches the age at which milk is not the substantial part of her diet, her choice may be to eat nothing, particularly if the choices on the tray are not to her liking. If she doesn't want to eat, she shouldn't be forced to. A child who recognizes early on that food is provided to answer hunger—that it is not a reward or a source of conflict—will eat when hungry.

The parents, however, should remain in complete control of the choices to be offered. This control persists until nursery school or kindergarten. Of course, a baby-sitter or relative may intervene at times. If so, the parents have to take pains to inform the well-meaning interloper what they want the baby to eat and insist this diet be adhered to in a consistent manner.

As Elizabeth's ability to feed herself grows, neurodevelopment once again complements behavioral development. At first the feeding is, shall we say, less than elegant. Finger foods and what some mothers refer to as "face foods" end up everywhere. The parent with a desire to supervise too closely and control too tightly has to resist the urge to make sure baby doesn't make a mess. The mess is only in the eyes of the adult beholder. The infant is oblivious to and, in fact, may enjoy the mess. As the child grows and develops, the ability to make a mess takes on refinement. The child practices, awkwardly but finally expertly, using the two basic tools of the nutritional trade: the cup and spoon. Elizabeth, for example, drinks from a cup by a year of age and masters the spoon two to three months later. Only practice makes perfect, so she should be allowed and even encouraged to try feeding herself with both. Here Mrs. Richardson has to resist the temptation to do everything for her baby, who may, for a while at least, seem to want only to be spoon-fed. Elizabeth really needs to develop her independence—it is, after all, inevitable.

As Elizabeth becomes more mobile in her environment, she is able to forage farther afield for new foodstuffs. Some caution must be exercised here, since "foodstuffs" to the toddler may include dirt, paint chips, turpentine, and medications of all sorts. Ingestion of such nonfoods is called "pica." Pica reaches its peak in the two- to three-year-old age group. It does not affect all children, but those it does may incur toxic lead poisoning (from leaded paint chips in old buildings) and other accidental poisonings (from paint thinners to phenothiazines). No such materials are safe from the reach of the inquisitive toddler. Strict precautions must be taken to keep them out of the child's environment, by locking them in a childproof cabinet if necessary. It is to our shame that some 600,000 accidental poison ingestions occur each year.

Once the child has mastered the spoon and the cup and has achieved full mobility and balance, it is time for a change in the nutritional arena: away with the high chair in the kitchen and on to the chair at the dining room table. For most kids, this happens at about three to four years and represents a major event in the socialization process. It may also present problems which must be faced and solved by the entire family. With both parents present the chances for contradictions to be transmitted to the child are increased.

I know one particularly successful parent who ascribes her success in the transition from high chair to family table to three rules: (1) maintain a consistent approach, (2) never offer an alternative you cannot or are not willing to follow through with, and (3) never use food as a reward. Outbursts of pea throwing at the table are met with calmness. Her boy is asked to leave the table and come back when he's ready to use food for nutrition and not ballistics. When he chooses to come back, which, she says, normally does not take long, his dinner resumes, including dessert. At times, she admits, she has lost her temper at his misbehavior. She once threatened to drop a birthday cake out the window, but hastily took back her threat when she realized she wasn't prepared to follow through with it. Her own mother, she says, used to encourage her to eat her vegetables by offering her more chocolate, ice cream, cookies, and the like for every spoonful of vegetables. This using food as a reward, she's convinced, is why she now overeats whenever she gets depressed.

Up to this point in our discussion of the child's nutritional needs, the parents have been the sole providers of the child's diet. They have provided a balanced diet, based on their knowledge of nutritional values and of the developmental capabilities of their child. Now, however, the nutritional baton is about to be passed to other directors, at least for a considerable portion of the child's day. The nutritional ties that bind are, alas, about to be further loosened.

CHAPTER 8

Your Child's Nutrition: From School Time Through Adolescence

Changes in Nutritional Patterns with Growing Independence

By the time a child goes to school, it is safe to say that eating habits have been pretty well established. What changes particularly now is the source of the child's food. New caretakers come on the scene. The parents are no longer the sole providers of the child's nutrition. Although at first the school experience may be only a half-day long, it still means that the morning snack is prepared by someone other than mother or father. Gradually, as the child moves from kindergarten to first grade, or as the school experience becomes day-long, the snack is not the only nutritional experience supervised by the new caretakers—lunch is also served away from home. Lunch may be brought by the child to school or, if the child is attending a neighborhood school, it may continue to be served at home. But only in the second case will parents continue to supervise its consumption.

Once the student gets into the higher grades, the child may have to go farther from home to attend school. Lunch at home may no longer be an option. The child can still, of course, bring home-prepared lunch to school. If not, the child eats the lunch provided by the school cafeteria.

In federally funded school lunch programs, the kinds and amounts of food are based on the needs of ten- to twelve-year-old children and are varied in portion and size to meet the needs of other age groups. The type A lunch, as it is called, is designed to provide one-third of the daily nutritional needs and is made up of meat or meat alternatives, two or more fruits and/or vegetables, milk, and bread.

The other major change that occurs in the nutritional pattern of children in school is the eating environment: a large cafeteria in the presence of many other children. Parents should not be surprised when children come home with new nutritional ideas and tastes. "Harold's mother doesn't make him eat that." "Susan's lunch always has chocolate cookies."

I remember sharing lunchroom space with certain well-chosen friends whose mothers always provided Oreos and chocolate milk, since my mother refused to have those "sweets" in the house. Children beginning kindergarten at five years of age may be naive about such matters. After first grade they become seasoned professionals at scrounging forbidden foods. The ability to acquire food not offered at home increases even more in adolescence, when a part-time job may provide independent wealth to be expended on anything, even food. And no one, not even mom and dad, need know anything about it.

The reasons for pointing out these changes in eating pattern are twofold: to underline the importance of inculcating good eating habits in the years before school begins, and to help the parent accept and cope with loss of nutritional control over the child during time spent away from home. Two important meals, however, remain in the parental domain—breakfasts and dinners.

The Importance of Breakfast

Breakfast is an important meal for many reasons. Blood sugar levels are lowest in the morning after a night without food. (In fact, in the diagnosis of diabetes mellitus, a disease in which blood sugar levels may remain unusually high, tests are made before breakfast, when the individual's blood sugar should normally be at its lowest.) A normal breakfast causes two major metabolic events to occur: blood sugar levels go up, giving the child energy for the day; and insulin is released, guaranteeing that sugar present in excess will be stored in the liver and muscles as glycogen or in the fat cells as fat. Energy, in either case, will be available for later in the day. Because starches are complex carbohydrates, they take longer to raise the sugar level and so do not excite as sudden an insulin release. For this reason, some nutritionists feel that starches (such as cereals and breads) allow for a more gradual and prolonged provision of energy. Without breakfast, the child's first meal is lunch. Allowing for at least one hour after meals for blood sugar levels to be significantly elevated, if a child eats lunch between 12:00 and 1:00 P.M., it will be two o'clock, close to the time the child is ready to come home from school, before the energy lift needed for the day is received.

Another important nutrient often lost if breakfast is missed is vitamin C. By convention, breakfast in America has become the meal at which fruits and fruit juices are mainly, if not exclusively, provided. The child under eleven years old needs roughly 45 milligrams a day of vitamin C in order to maintain adequate reserves of that vitamin and to replace the amount metabolized daily by the body. Children over eleven have the same 60 milligrams per day requirement that adults have.

"Excuse me for interrupting," said Mrs. Richardson when I spoke to her about the vitamin C requirements of her daughter

Elizabeth, who was now in the first grade. "Can you translate that into apples and oranges?"

"One average size apple contains slightly more than 75 milligrams of vitamin C. One average size orange has 70 milligrams. Three ounces of freshly squeezed orange juice has 45 milligrams of vitamin C. One half of a grapefruit has close to 75 milligrams."

"What is vitamin C good for, except preventing colds?" she asked.

"First of all, it has never been proved that vitamin C will prevent colds. About ten years ago, Nobel Prize winner Linus Pauling contended that taking large amounts of vitamin C—more than 1,000 milligrams per day—would reduce the frequency and severity of symptoms of the common cold. However, other scientists found no clear difference in frequency or severity of colds in people who were given vitamin C and people who were given a placebo—that is, the equivalent of a sugar tablet. The 1980 *Recommended Dietary Allowance* reported that 'the benefits of large doses of ascorbic acid are too small to justify recommending routine intakes of large amounts for the entire population.' We also know that 80 to 90 percent of vitamin C is absorbed if the daily intake is less than 100 milligrams a day, but that less of the vitamin is absorbed if more than this is taken.

"All of this is not to say that vitamin C is not important. We do know that vitamin C deficiency can cause scurvy and is also associated with impaired wound healing. Scurvy is a potentially fatal disease causing weakening of the walls of capillaries, the small blood vessels that form a lacework connection between arteries and veins. When the capillary walls weaken, they rupture easily, leading to extensive hemorrhaging in the body."

"How awful," said Mrs. Richardson.

"Awful, indeed, but fortunately quite rare in this country. In pediatrics we see it only in infants raised exclusively on cow's milk, or in infants breast-fed by mothers whose own stores of the vitamin have been depleted because of severely limited diets."

"I remember you said that breast milk has vitamin C but cow's milk does not. Why don't baby calves get scurvy, then?"

"Vitamin C is present in unpasteurized cow's milk, which is what the calf receives, but the heat necessary for pasteurization inactivates it. That's why although tomatoes, potatoes, and leafy vegetables contain vitamin C, these vegetables may not be good sources of the vitamin if they are overcooked.

"There is another important feature of the balanced breakfast, particularly regarding vitamin C and iron. If the vitamin C content of the meal is 25 to 75 milligrams or more, iron absorption is improved. This means that if eggs are taken along with an orange or orange juice, for instance, the availability of iron provided by the egg yolk will be enhanced. This is not to say that breakfast needs to be the only source of vitamin C. It would be healthful for Elizabeth if you'd give her fruit to take to school, or if you'd serve it as dessert at dinner. Nor am I making a testimonial for eggs at breakfast every day. Eggs three to four times a week should be enough—even for people who are not particularly cholesterol conscious. Just don't forget that eggs are a very nutritious food and should not be totally excluded from the diet."

"So for breakfast," Mrs. Richardson said, "I continue to provide the same balanced diet for Elizabeth that I do for my husband and myself. For lunch, I pack her off to school with a sandwich, usually meat with some lettuce or a tomato slice, a piece of fruit, and some cookies. She buys milk at school. Is there any special advice about dinner?" she asked.

"No. But remember that as she gets older, dinner may be the one meal you all end up sharing together. In fact, national averages show that by age seventeen, only half our children eat more than one meal at home."

The Adolescent's Nutritional Needs

The above bit of information signals that it is now time to step away from our concentration on the parent-provider and focus our attention more clearly on the adolescent.

Adolescence cannot be precisely defined by chronological age. Our common chronological concept of adolescents as "teenagers" is erroneous, since either males or females may begin their pubertal metamorphosis as early as eight to ten years of age. Nutritional needs are directly related to the adolescent growth spurt, the greatest burst of growth that the child will experience aside from growth during infancy. Since the growth spurt is integrally related to other changes in adolescence, and since these changes differ so much between the sexes, it is important to review them before setting down nutritional guidelines for this period. For this reason also, we must now discuss boys and girls separately. The ages given in our discussion for onset of each pubertal event are only approximations. As we will see, the sexual maturity of the adolescent boy or girl is of much greater use in predicting nutritional needs than chronological maturity.

The normal growth of pubic hair and progression of breast development in girls and growth of pubic hair and genitalia in males were described by an English doctor, J. M. Tanner. He assigned a number to each of the milestones in the development of the secondary sexual difference. The numbers, given in Roman numerals I to V, are called "Tanner stages." Males and females progress along a regular sequence from Tanner stage I, which is prepubescence, to Tanner stage V, which is adulthood. Each girl is scored separately for pubic hair and for breast development, and each boy separately for pubic hair and for development of the genitals. This is done because of the different rates of development of these sexual characteristics. For example, a girl may be at Tanner stage II for breast development and still be at Tanner stage I for pubic hair development.

The adolescent girl gets off to an earlier start than the boy both in her sexual maturation and in her growth spurt. For the girl, the growth spurt begins, on the average, at eight to ten years, usually a year before any changes in sexual characteristics have begun. The rate of height growth reaches its peak (called the "peak height velocity") when she is roughly twelve years old. This is two years earlier than it occurs in boys. Approximately a year after she has achieved her peak height velocity, menstruation (menarche) occurs. The onset and rate of sexual maturation, and menarche itself, are apparently affected by the weight of the child. Fatter children on the whole start maturation and achieve menarche earlier than their thinner counterparts. Children who are severely undernourished develop their secondary sexual characteristics later. The tendency for children today to develop secondary sexual characteristics earlier than in previous generations and the general decrease in the average age of menarche might be related to overall improved nutrition of the population.

In any case, peak height velocity occurs and is already beginning to decelerate before menarche. By the time peak height velocity occurs, the adolescent girl is already somewhere between Tanner stage III and IV, both for breast and for pubic hair development. Her breasts will have the appearance of small adult breasts, but she will still be a couple of years away from reaching the Tanner V adult stage. The entire process of moving from Tanner I to Tanner V takes an average of four and one half years, but it cannot be overstressed that this and the other chronological statistics are only averages. One difficulty in dealing with maturation of the adolescent child is that one must always take into account the wide range of individual variation within what is considered normal.

Whereas the adolescent girl reaches the peak of her growth spurt well before the completion of her secondary sexual development, the average male is almost a Tanner V before his growth spurt reaches its peak. On average, the male's peak occurs around two years after the female has achieved hers. It is obvious, then, that nutritional planning for the adolescent boys in a junior high school class, say, should be considerably different from that for the girls in the same class.

There are other significant differences in the maturation of boys and girls. Although growth begins earlier in girls, their rate of growth is less than the rate of growth for boys, with girls achieving less of a total increase in height than boys. Boys also gain more weight than girls and they do it faster, and as they do there is a change in distribution of body weight. The proportions of fat and lean body mass (weight made up of muscle and skeletal tissue) are roughly the same in boys and girls before the onset of puberty. During puberty boys gain more weight in the form of lean body mass while losing fat. Girls show growth in fat and muscle to the extent that when they have completed adolescence they will have about twice as much body fat as boys and one-half the muscle mass. These figures are based on studies done in this country in the early 1970s and are not, to my knowledge, cross-cultural; nor, of course, do they take into account the recent increase in athletics for girls.

"You'd *better* add that," said Janet, a twelve-and-a-half-year-old who had been quietly listening while I talked to her parents about adolescent growth. Janet was a swimmer who had been competing since she was ten years old. She had a physique that was distinctly more lean body mass than fat. "I'm not so fat," she added.

"I was just talking about national averages," I said. "An average is just an average. You're exceptional."

"I was only kidding," she said. "I'm actually really interested in nutrition and food and was paying attention to what you were saying. I understand the differences between girls and boys—I mean as far as their growth is concerned. We learned a lot of that in health class. Let's say I was average—you know, not counting the workouts—what should I be eating now?"

Janet was about a Tanner IV in her sexual maturation, by

my estimate, and just reaching her peak height velocity. If this was indeed the case, her nutritional needs for growth at this stage would be at their maximum.

"If you were average, you'd need about 2,500 calories a day. Do you know what calories are?"

"Sure," she said. She glanced at her parents. "Mom and Dad are always counting them. They say if they eat too many calories they'll get fat. Is 2,500 calories more or less than my mother is eating?"

"I've no way of knowing, unless she wants to tell me." I smiled at Janet's mother. "But she's probably eating about 1,000 calories less than that each day, if she's trying not to gain weight."

"The difference is that I'm growing still," Janet said. "That's why I need to eat more, like you said."

"That's right, and we haven't taken into account the calories you need for your exercise."

"So how do I know how much I should be eating?" she asked.

"Trust your appetite. For now, eat when you're hungry. In another couple of years or so you'll be finished with your rapid growth spurt. You'll probably continue to grow until you're twenty or so, but in the meantime, your growth rate will be slowing down. So, as the years pass, don't . . ."

"Keep eating so much or I'll get fat," she finished.

"That's right. You won't need to eat as much."

"What about my brother Robert?" she asked. Janet's brother was four years older than she and also an athlete. He had been running on his high school's cross-country team since he was fifteen. He was now sixteen and just finishing his growth spurt. According to the national estimate, his daily energy requirements would be about 3,000 calories. The need for calories for growth alone would be beginning to taper off. The 3,000-calorie figure, however, does not take into account Robert's extra requirements for his athletic endeavors.

Both children require sufficient protein to take care of their energy expenditure. Proteins should form 10 to 15 percent of their calories. Boys, on the average, require more protein intake because of their relatively greater muscle mass. They also have a greater requirement for iron, since their blood volume expands along with their muscle mass. But once a girl has begun to menstruate, her iron needs will become much the same as a boy's. Adolescents in general tend not to eat enough iron and should be encouraged to eat more iron-containing foods, such as red meats, dried beans, green vegetables, and iron-fortified cereal products. Simultaneous increase in their vitamin C (ascorbic acid) intake from fruits and raw vegetables will help them absorb the iron contained in sources other than meat.

"Do I need to be taking vitamins?" asked Janet.

"Not if you're eating a balanced diet," I said. "And that includes meats, vegetables, whole grains such as bread and cereals, and fruits."

Recent large-scale nutritional surveys in this country have shown that specific vitamin deficiencies are not prevalent among adolescents. Vitamins A, B_6, C, and folic acid intakes are less than the recommended level in some adolescent populations, particularly in low income groups, but serious deficiency states have not been found. Rather than prescribe vitamins, I recommend the following foods to assure these nutrients are at the recommended level:

Dark yellow and dark green leafy vegetables for vitamin A.
Whole grain cereals, seeds, nuts, legumes, potatoes, meats, and fish for vitamin B_6.
Citrus fruits and juices for vitamin C.
Citrus fruits and dark green leafy vegetables for folic acid.

Once again, an increase in calories of a balanced diet will provide the required vitamins as well.

"Mother says I should drink more milk," said Janet. "But I don't like it that much. My brother does, though."

Calcium, which is provided in good quantity in milk and cheese, is necessary for good skeletal growth. Boys need more calcium than girls because of their increased skeletal growth during puberty. Calcium is a very important mineral for the body. When combined with phosphorus, it forms the soft center of the bone that will later harden (calcify) to form the sturdy but flexible shaft that supports weight and serves as an anchor to tendons and muscles. Calcium in the blood, as opposed to bone calcium, is also extremely important but present in lesser quantities. This calcium is necessary for blood coagulation, for function of the heart muscle, and for contraction of other muscles in the body. These functions are so important for survival that we have evolved highly sensitive ways to maintain the blood concentration of calcium, ways so sensitive that the level never varies in a healthy person more than 3 percent in either direction from the norm. This concentration is maintained through hormonal control of absorption and excretion in the intestinal tract and kidneys, and through absorption or deposit of calcium in the bones.

"You mean my bones are always changing?" asked Janet. "Come on. A bone is a bone."

"You're right on both counts," I said. "A bone is a bone, but it is always changing. Our bones are no different from the various organs in our body. They are alive and growing. Furthermore, bones serve as the storage reservoirs for the important minerals in our bodies—calcium, magnesium, and phosphorus. When your body needs more calcium, it takes some from the bone. When it needs less, it puts more back into the bone."

Since the composition of bone is a complex containing calcium and phosphorus bound together, the amount of calcium that gets deposited in bone is influenced by the amount of absorbed and circulating phosphate or phosphorus. It's like mixing glue and resin together to form epoxy cement: the two have to be deposited together or they won't stick. If there is too much phosphorus around, calcium is removed from the circulation and deposited in bone. Low phosphorus favors movement of calcium from bone into the circulation.

Another part of the process has already been described in our discussion of the calcium requirement of pregnant mothers who drank a lot of phosphorus-containing soft drinks: too much phosphorus in the diet interferes with the absorption of calcium from the intestines. It may also be that too much protein in the diet increases calcium excretion in the kidneys. We do know that a measurable amount of calcium is lost in sweat, even if the body is low in calcium to begin with.

So with all of these factors—rapid skeletal growth, the potentially high phosphorus intake of adolescents who drink a lot of soda, the increased protein intake needed during the growth spurt, and the adolescent's increased physical activity leading to sweating and calcium loss—we have ample reasons for insisting that adolescent children get plenty of calcium and, because it assures the efficient absorption of calcium from the intestines, plenty of vitamin D as well. The latter most kids get simply by spending a lot of time outdoors. They will also get plenty if they drink fortified milk as their calcium source. Most adolescents don't get the recommended dietary allowances for calcium intake in their diets. And yet they do not develop rickets or other signs of calcium deficiency. Many of them are like Janet, who doesn't like milk. Why they are spared from ill effects is unclear. It may be that they are not, that their growth is impaired by their reduced calcium and vitamin D intake and that they would actually be taller if they ingested more of these nutrients. The recommended allowances are, as we know, set high to guarantee adequate intake by all members of the population. It is also known that calcium is absorbed more efficiently when the intake is low.

"So I don't need to drink my milk?" asked Janet.

"That's not the point. You need all the calcium you can get. Drink your milk, and eat cheese, too. It can be skim milk if you like, but don't run the risk of interfering with your growth just because you don't like milk. You also get magnesium in milk, which is another important mineral for normal nerve and muscle activity."

"You make it all sound so scary," she said, "like I should walk around counting calories, counting calcium, magnesium, everything."

"I'm sorry. I don't want to scare you at all. You don't have to go around counting anything. It's just that sometimes it's tempting to try out new diets that aren't well balanced. Or sometimes you get hooked on a single food and its all you want to eat. That's the only time I get scared. Too much of any one thing in your diet when you're growing fast and exercising a lot isn't good. That's when imbalances occur that can make you sick or interfere with your growth. Whereas, if you eat some meat, vegetables, fruits, and cheese and drink milk—as much of them as you want—throughout every week, you'll be healthy and do well."

"How about for my swimming?" Janet asked. "Robert asked me to ask you if he and I should be taking extra vitamins for our sports. He's a runner, you know."

"The claim that extra vitamins will help you in your athletic performance isn't true. And the idea about eating a lot of protein to give you energy before a race isn't true either."

"It isn't? But the coach told me I should have steak the night before each meet, that it would set me up with energy for the race. Robert's coach told him to eat spaghetti. We had a big fight with Mom when we both had a race the next day. She finally told us to cook our own meals."

Nutrition for Exercise

Proper nutrition for exercise is of great importance for the athletic adolescent. Among younger children, those less than five years old particularly, the marginally undernourished will automatically reduce their physical activity in order to allow their limited supply of available energy to be channeled into growth. Adolescents are different. With peer pressure, parental pressure, and frequent pressure from overcompetitive coaches exhorting kids to ever-greater heights of athletic performance, adolescents are tempted to ignore the various danger signals transmitted by their bodies indicating potential growth or health problems.

In order to understand better the nutritional needs of the adolescent athlete, let's review the way the body produces energy under various conditions and stresses as well as the way this energy output can be measured. Since Janet's brother Robert is an athlete and is participating in long-distance running in which energy output can be measured (speed and distance measured in time and miles), let's follow him through a workout and apply our understanding of energy metabolism to his actual performance.

In order for the body to produce energy for its work, it needs two things: oxygen and fuel. The gasoline-driven engine is an obvious analogy here. (We even talk about burning up energy, and, in fact, as we exercise we do produce heat.) Reduction in either the oxygen or the fuel will cause reduction in the efficiency of our car's engine. Similar reduction does the same thing to energy production in the body.

But, of course, human beings are not combustion engines. For one thing, we can produce energy for short periods of time without oxygen, as in anaerobic exercise. Production of energy in anaerobic exercise is not as efficient as production in aerobic exercise, for which oxygen is required. Anaerobic exercise can go on for only a short time before its available sources of energy are used up. In addition, when we exercise anaerobically we produce more lactic acid, and large amounts of lactic acid can further limit our ability to exercise over longer periods of time. One example of anaerobic exercise is the 100-yard dash in track—another is the 20-yard dash to catch a bus. What makes the dash anaerobic is not that some sprinters, and bus chasers, don't breathe while they run, but that the burst of exercise places such a sudden demand for energy on the body that it doesn't have time to deliver to the muscles that are exercising the oxygen necessary for aerobic metabolism. If we start off slower and give our body time to provide the oxygen necessary for our exercise, we will not use up our full supply nearly so fast and will consequently be able to go on for a much longer time.

So we see that prolonged exercise requires the delivery of oxygen to the exercising muscles. If we can efficiently provide oxygen to the muscles, we are in good shape. If we're in good shape, we can walk for miles, or run a considerable distance, or climb up a couple of flights of stairs and hardly be out of breath. That's because our body is so good at providing oxygen to the muscles that it doesn't have to make us breathe harder during these minimal exercises in order to provide more. On the other hand, we all know what it's like to be out of shape.

We take in oxygen through our lungs. In the lungs it gets transferred to the hemoglobin in the blood that circulates through the lungs just to pick up the oxygen. The oxygen is then delivered by the blood to all of our tissues, since they all need oxygen to live. But it goes "special delivery," so to speak, to the exercising muscle, which registers a temporary but emphatic need for more energy. In the exercising muscle it is used for the aerobic metabolism of fuel, thus producing energy. The fuels metabolized are the familiar ones—fats, carbohydrates, and protein.

Anything that improves our ability to deliver oxygen puts us in better shape: the capacity or volume of our lungs; the amount of hemoglobin in our blood available to pick up the oxygen and carry it throughout the body; the efficiency of our circulation—that is, our heart and arteries and veins—in delivering the oxygen quickly to where it is needed. You'll note that breathing faster is not included in this list. Breathing faster is an inefficient way of increasing our oxygen uptake. It is inefficient because the harder and faster we breathe, the more energy our muscles of respiration consume. Our body's responding to increased oxygen need by increasing our respiratory rate is important for survival, but it cannot be taken as a sign of being in good shape.

All of this physiological background can help us understand an important test used in exercise physiology to study fitness. That test is called the "maximum oxygen uptake test" and measures the maximum amount of oxygen that a person can take in over a period of time. This amount is abbreviated "VO_2 max" (V standing for volume, O_2 for oxygen, and max for maximum). The test is given in a laboratory, where a person either pedals a bicycle or runs on a treadmill while breathing a measurable amount of oxygen through a mouthpiece. Gradually, the treadmill is put on an incline and goes a bit faster, or a brake is applied to the bicycle and the subject has to pedal against it. As the work load increases, the body's demands for energy and oxygen increase, and the subject responds by breathing faster and more deeply. The heart rate increases to pump blood faster throughout the body. More and more oxygen is taken up by the body. Finally, however, a limit is reached. We are, after all, mortals. We all come to a point at which, despite the fact that our bodies may cry out for more energy, we cannot take up any more oxygen. This point is called the VO_2 max. Once we've reached our VO_2 max, our bodies switch to non-oxygen (anaerobic) metabolism, which, as we pointed out, is inefficient and will rapidly burn up whatever fuel supply we have left. Exhaustion is right around the corner. Obviously, the higher our VO_2 max, the better shape we are in.

Not all exercise, of course, is "all out." In fact, for a variety of complex reasons, we ordinarily do not perform at our maximum oxygen uptake for very long. In everyday life, we operate below our VO_2 max, and the percentage of VO_2 max we do operate on determines, as we shall see, what fuel we use. The fuel sources are different for the pedestrian and the driver; they are different for the athlete and the sedentary person. Understanding the fuels that are being used in our various expenditures of energy will help us decide what foods should be taken in.

Janet's brother's high school is located about one mile from the track where he begins his after-school workouts. A bus goes there, but Robert feels a certain pride in being a long-distance runner, so he walks to practice everyday. (He also walks to and from school.)

When Robert walks, he goes at a brisk pace. He's hardly aware of this fact unless he's walking with friends who are not in as good condition as he is. His brisk pace puts him at about 20 to 30 percent of his VO_2 max. His friends might be at about 35 percent of their VO_2 max, depending on how fast they are going and how badly out of shape they are. Because of his conditioning, he could keep going at this pace for hours. The limiting factor would not be his oxygen uptake. He is taking in oxygen very efficiently and with no trouble whatsoever. The limiting factors would be fuel and water.

At low to moderate levels of exercise (30 percent of VO_2 max), the primary fuel for energy is fat, although carbohydrates are also being used in the form of glycogen. Fat, you will recall, is the storage form of energy in the body. A molecule of fat is capable of producing two and a half times as much energy as a molecule of glycogen, the major carbohydrate energy source. Per ounce, fat has three times as much energy as glycogen, since each molecule of glycogen is stored with a considerable amount of water. An ounce of fat is pure fat, whereas an ounce of glycogen is part carbohydrate and part water. So fat has the advantage of being a very efficient form of stored energy. Its disadvantages are that it can be metabolized to produce energy only in the presence of oxygen, its metabolism takes a long time compared to glycogen's, and it requires more oxygen for its metabolism than glycogen. Glycogen is rapidly metabolized with or without oxygen.

This means that if Robert is exercising at a low percentage of his VO_2 max, at which oxygen can be provided easily and in abundance and at which it does not have to be provided too quickly, fat is the ideal source of energy. The reason he can go on and on at his brisk pace is that the body's supply of fat, even in relatively lean individuals, is almost limitless. (An obese individual on a starvation diet can go months without any major caloric intake as long as there is an adequate supply of water available.)

Once Robert has arrived at the track, he changes into his running clothes and does his warmup stretching exercises. He is still functioning at considerably less than 50 percent of his maximum oxygen uptake and still metabolizing fats predominantly. The coach tells him that today's workout will be a "time trial" (intra-team race) to see who will be traveling to the state championship.

The race will be five miles, longer than Robert has raced before. As he stands on the starting line, his adrenaline release is making his heart go faster. He's also beginning to breathe a little faster, because of the adrenaline and because his increased heart rate is already requiring more oxygen.

"On your mark, get set . . ." and the starting gun goes off! Robert jumps to an early lead. At this point, his body is producing energy without consuming oxygen. He is *anaerobically* metabolizing glycogen because the sudden demand of the muscles for energy temporarily overtakes the ability of the body to deliver oxygen. After he gets into a good position, he settles into a more comfortable pace. The race will take between thirty and forty minutes, and he has been running for a little more than two. Now his body has a chance to provide oxygen to his muscles. His body now also starts metabolizing glycogen more efficiently—that is, more energy is released for every molecule of glycogen metabolized. He feels better. The oxygen arriving at his muscles gives him the ability to function aerobically, which gives him his "second" wind. He settles comfortably into second place. He is now running at approximately 70 percent of his VO_2 max, and his body is almost exclusively metabolizing glycogen. The race winds through a park, over some hills. His breathing actually becomes more steady than it was at the beginning of the race. He maintains an even pace at 70 percent of his maximum oxygen uptake. At this pace, his body begins to metabolize fats, but this comparatively slow process won't have its full effect until he is twenty minutes into the race.

If Robert were running a marathon (technically 26 miles, 385 yards), his body would continue to metabolize fats long into the race. And the metabolism of this energy source would keep his body from using up its more easily exhausted glycogen supplies, which are stored in the liver and in muscle. When a runner's glycogen stores are exhausted, the race is in fact over, whether or not the finish line has been reached. In a shorter race, one less than an hour long, the glycogen stores will not be used up as readily, so metabolism of fat as a glycogen-sparing phenomenon is not as important.

Robert is now nearing the last half-mile of the race. He is still in second place. The third-place runner is far behind. The leader of the race is a senior named Jerry, not a bad guy but someone he's always wanted to beat. Jerry is about 20 yards ahead of him. Robert can catch him in one of two ways. He can sprint up to his side, covering the 20 yards in a few seconds. This tactic would be time saving, but energy inefficient. Sprinting at this point would mean more anaerobic metabolism, caused by demands for sudden energy for which the body cannot supply oxygen. His body would burn up a lot of glycogen, maybe most of what it has left, and produce lactic acid— all of which would get him to Jerry's side, but no farther. What about the remaining half-mile or so? Or, instead of the fast sprint, Robert could gauge the distance left in the race and time his move accordingly. He could gradually increase his pace, pushing himself closer to 90 percent of his VO_2 max as he narrows the distance between himself and his rival. No anaerobic metabolism, no lactic acid production. And still something left when Robert catches his opponent.

Robert wisely decides on the second plan. Keeping an eye

on Jerry, he increases his pace gradually. He sees the finish line 100 yards off as he catches up with the front-runner and starts to pass him. But Jerry isn't willing simply to let him go by. Both runners accelerate until, with 50 yards left, they're sprinting to the finish line. Neck and neck, all out. Now it's pure anaerobic metabolism and buildup of lactic acid for both. Now the one with the extra glycogen will win as the supply dwindles in the final yards. Jerry falters just two strides from the finish line. Robert's body strains to extract the last grams of glycogen from his muscles, and he wins the race.

This discussion of the physiology of Robert's victory puts us in a better position to discuss his nutritional needs as an athlete. Two things are striking: the importance of carbohydrates as the major source of energy, and the unimportance of protein. Protein, you will notice, was never mentioned in our discussion of the race.

"So I don't need protein while I'm in training, then?" asked Robert, who had dropped by my office at the urging of his sister to discuss the nutritional needs created by his running.

"That's not the point. You certainly do need protein, but for cell growth, not for energy. And if you increase the amount of food you eat each day in order to get more energy calories for your running, you'll also get more protein."

Robert looked confused, so we sat down with a pencil and paper and made a few calculations.

Robert needs 3,000 calories a day for normal growth, 10 to 12 percent of which should come from protein, 35 to 40 percent from fats, and 48 to 50 percent from carbohydrates. This means 75 grams a day of protein, 133 grams of fat, and 342 grams of carbohydrates. He needs at least an additional 1,500 calories each day for his running, but here the proportion of fats, carbohydrates, and proteins will be different. For these additional calories, the proportion of carbohydrates should be higher because of their importance in exercise. Fats exist in considerable quantity in the body to begin with, so there should be no need for adding more. Protein will not be necessary for energy, but it will be for increase in lean body mass, not, however, in an amount significantly above what he is already taking. We can answer all of Robert's needs by dividing the 1,500 additional calories like so: 52 percent carbohydrates, 35 percent fats (same as before), and 13 percent protein. His proper diet, which combines the 3,000 calories for growth and the 1,500 for athletics, will amount to roughly 135 grams protein, 180 grams fats, and 550 grams carbohydrates. Robert will get more protein by increasing the caloric intake of his diet, but the most striking aspect of his diet is its increased carbohydrate content.

"So I need to eat more calories, and a lot of my food should be carbohydrates," said Robert. "Sugar is a carbohydrate. So that means more sweets. Great!"

"More calories, and a lot of carbohydrates, but *not* more sugar," I corrected him. "Sugar is okay within limits. We talk about it providing 'empty calories,' which means it provides calories only—no vitamins or minerals. If sedentary people eat more sugar they get nothing out of it but more fat. Remember, excess calories go into fat. You are in the enviable position of exercising so much each day that all those extra calories will be used, not stored. However," I added, "you also have an increased need for vitamins and minerals, which are contained in foods that have more complex carbohydrates, such as potatoes, grains, pasta, and so on. I recommend taking most of your carbohydrates in that form."

"How do I know how much to eat?" Robert asked. His sister had asked the same question, and my answer to Robert was the same as my answer to Janet.

"Follow your appetite. It's still the best gauge of your nutritional needs. Don't eat when you're not hungry or just for something to do. And remember one thing: if you stop training, you also have to cut back on your calories."

The calculations for Robert's diet would be roughly the same for any adolescent participating in formal athletics. Carbohydrates are needed in greater quantity, and protein will be provided as the calories taken in are increased. This kind of ongoing diet will sustain a high degree of daily exercise.

As we continued talking, Robert asked some questions about his particular athletic interest: racing. What to eat the night before a race? What to eat the morning of a race? What to eat or drink during a marathon race?

"I've heard a lot about something called the 'carbohydrate loading diet,' " he said. "Isn't that where you eat nothing but carbohydrates before a race?"

"Well, yes," I replied. "But it's more complicated than that. It's a highly specific diet for competitive events that require sustained exercise for more than an hour or so. Long-distance running, cross-country skiing, bicycle racing would all fit into this category. These are all events where the amount of glycogen you have in your muscles may be the performance-limiting factor."

"No glycogen—no go," he said. "Isn't that what marathon runners call 'hitting the wall'?"

The term "hitting the wall" refers to a point in a marathon, usually around the 20-mile mark, where runners literally feel themselves run out of energy. Some people contend that it happens only to less accomplished runners and that it has more to do with the amount of time run than the actual distance, since the amount of calories burned up is more dependent on the total time run than on the speed of the run. A runner completing each mile of a marathon in 7 minutes might "hit the wall" when he or she completes 20 miles after 2½ hours. Elite distance runners complete the race in 2 hours and 10 minutes, which may be one reason they don't "hit the wall."

Physiologically, this uncomfortable and discouraging phenomenon is believed to represent the complete exhaustion of glycogen stores in the muscles and the liver. It happens unexpectedly—like suddenly coming up against a brick wall. The runner may be feeling quite strong at 18 miles and then, a mile later, feel dizzy, weak, and suddenly incapable of moving another foot.

Researchers in Sweden did muscle biopsies of long-distance runners and detected a measurable depletion of glycogen in runners who "hit the wall." This finding has led them to equate the ability to do well in a marathon with the amount of glycogen left in the muscle tissue. Researchers have also demonstrated that the amount of muscle glycogen can be increased by dietary changes—by what has come to be called the "carbohydrate loading diet."

To profit from this diet, the runner must first deplete the muscles of glycogen as completely as possible. This can be accomplished in one of two ways. The runner can start on the regimen six days before the race (a race longer than 10 to 15 miles). On day one, the runner goes 10 to 15 miles at a very fast pace. This uses up most of the available muscle glycogen. For two and three days, the runner continues to work out but eats a low-carbohydrate diet, consuming almost all calories as fats or protein. This process should totally eliminate any glycogen from the muscle or liver. The other way of accomplishing depletion is by doing a 20- to 25-mile run on the same day carbohydrate loading is started. However, since carbohydrate loading begins only three days before the race, most athletes feel this method to be too exhausting.

Apparently, when glycogen depletion is accomplished, the enzymes used to manufacture glycogen from any source begin to work overtime, so to speak. There is no running for three days prior to the race. During this time, the runner consumes a diet of normal calories made up almost entirely of carbohydrates. This is the actual "carbohydrate loading," and the end result, shown by biochemical analysis of muscle biopsies, is an increase of two to three times the normal amount of glycogen in the muscle. Both Swedish researchers and researchers in the U.S. have shown that there is a good correlation between this increase in muscle glycogen and the length of time an athlete can sustain maximal performance.

"Why doesn't everybody use the diet?" asked Robert.

"Apparently everybody doesn't need it, and certainly everybody doesn't like it," I answered. "The ones who don't need it are the elite marathoners. It has been shown that the highly trained athlete is able to use enough fat during sustained athletic performance so that his or her glycogen will never go down to zero. Adding more doesn't help. In fact, it may hinder performance. And there are other reasons many runners don't like it. First, they don't like the way it makes them feel the week before a race. Those three days of depletion are miserable. The body is being deprived of sugar which it needs to function normally. Second, as you may remember, when glycogen is stored in the body it is stored with water. When the muscle glycogen stores are increased two- to threefold, the muscle feels heavier and stiffer because of all the added water weight. The carbohydrate loading diet has to be viewed as a very special diet to be used for a very special kind of athletic event. I don't recommend it. It seems to me that your body is under enough stress the week before a race. The diet just adds more."

"How does all this tie in with the pre-event dinner?" asked Robert.

"Knowledge of the metabolism of energy in any athletic event has helped us change our way of thinking about the pre-event dinner," I said. "It used to be steak and potatoes, with the emphasis on the steak. This was in the days when everyone in sports looked on protein as the only important food for the athlete. As we have seen in the physiological analysis of your time trial and in the research on carbohydrate loading, the most important foods are those containing carbohydrates. Complex carbohydrates taken in the night before will actually provide the bulk of energy needed for the event the next day."

"You mean my breakfast before the race isn't important?" asked Robert.

"Not so far as the race is concerned," I said. I then went on to explain why athletes should be careful about eating just prior to an event.

When we ingest carbohydrates, we increase our blood glucose level and stimulate the release of insulin, a hormone necessary for the uptake and metabolism of glucose in the muscles. Insulin is also important for promoting the storage of excessive glucose in the form of fats and glycogen. It also suppresses the release of glucose from the liver. By these pathways, insulin serves to reduce the elevated blood sugar. If there is a sudden demand for glucose (as in strenuous exercise) just when the insulin effect is reaching its peak, the blood glucose level can drop too far. The brain does not receive enough sugar, and the individual experiences the symptoms of hypoglycemia ("hypo" meaning low, "glycemia" meaning blood glucose): dizziness, exhaustion, and loss of consciousness.

"So I shouldn't have anything to eat just before my race," said Robert. "What is 'just before'?"

"About two hours is a safe limit," I said.

"Should a runner take in sugar during a long-distance race?" he asked.

"It's probably not helpful," I said. "And it may lead to an embarrassing complication: diarrhea. If you take in a high concentration of sugar, it can't all be absorbed, and what passes into the intestines draws water along with it. That's what can cause the diarrhea. Taking sugar in a lower concentration won't do that, but it probably won't do much to increase your energy, either."

I went on to explain to Robert that the most important thing to take during a long race or in any prolonged athletic event is water. During any strenuous exercise, the amount of water we lose by sweating and by breathing fast is considerable and must be replaced for normal body function and for the prevention of heat stroke. Heat stroke occurs when the body becomes so dehydrated it no longer has the ability to lose heat. The individual goes into shock, and the body temperature may go as high as 107 degrees Fahrenheit. This is a very dangerous and potentially life-threatening condition. Heat is a by-product of energy production—just as it is produced in the combustion engine we used as an analogy at the beginning of this section. Normally, in order to remove heat from the body we sweat, and as the sweat evaporates it cools off the body. On very hot and humid days the sweat does not evaporate as efficiently and we cannot lose heat as well. High temperatures and high humidity are dangerous for athletes because of the increased risk of heat stroke.

"Should I take salt tablets on those days?" asked Robert.

"No. You lose more water than salt in sweat. If you are eating a normal diet with the average amount of salt, you will maintain a normal salt balance. You may have to increase the foods containing potassium, however, since this is also lost in sweat. Eat more bananas and tomatoes."

Although we have concentrated on the runner in these pages on nutrition in athletics, the same precepts can be applied to any athletic endeavor. Sensitivity to the psychological and physiological needs of the growing athlete should be the goal of the school athletic program. The adolescent athlete should be groomed not merely to win, but, more importantly, to establish healthful patterns of regular exercise that can last throughout life. In my estimation, the success of any sport program is not to be gauged by its win-loss record but by the number of participants who will still be actively exercising in their thirties, forties, fifties, and even sixties and seventies. Knowledge of nutrition and how the body works can be a great help in achieving this goal as the young athlete learns respect for his or her growing body and is encouraged to give it the care it deserves.

PART II
Problems with Your Child's Nutrition

PART I of this book has offered some understanding of the mechanism of normal nutrition in the developing child. Although we have made occasional references to various problems and illnesses associated with poor nutrition, we have not been in a position to consider these abnormalities in detail until now. As in all medical education, a firm knowledge of what is normal is essential for recognizing, understanding, and treating what is not. The remainder of the book will be spent considering what is not normal. Topics will cover a range of problems, from very serious and life threatening to relatively benign and easily resolved. The intent is not to suggest that you accept the responsibility of being family doctor to your own children, but to help you become more alert to the early danger signals of a potentially serious problem and more reasonable in your approach to the more benign nutritional problems. This is, after all, the essence of health education.

Part II will deal with nutritional problems according to the age of the child. It is divided into three sections: the first year, toddler years to school age, and later years and adolescence. Some problems will, of course, arise at more than one age level. These have been included under the age level at which they are either most common or most serious. Failure to thrive is an example of such a problem. It is possible to find a child failing to thrive at any age, but it is more common and frequently more serious in the first year.

CHAPTER 9

Problems in the First Year

Failure to Thrive

FAILURE TO THRIVE is what most parents are really worried about in the first year. Almost every question about breast-feeding, choice of formula, frequency of feeding, amount, preferences, and so on is related to a lurking fear in every questioning parent's mind: is the baby growing all right? There's no denying it—normal growth is what it is all about, and failure to grow is failure to thrive.

To be more specific about the definition of failure to thrive, we have to look again at the growth chart. As mentioned before, a child whose growth can be plotted along the 5 percent line is growing normally along with 5 percent of other normal children. The fact that 95 percent of the population is taller or heavier does not make this child abnormal. Notice I said "taller" or "heavier." I did not say "growing faster." As long as growth follows that 5 percent curve, the child is growing at *approximately* the same rate as other children. By definition, this child is not failing to thrive.

Diagnosis of failure to thrive can be difficult. A parent named

[144]

Mrs. Lawrence brought in her three-month-old Adam because she was concerned that he wasn't growing. We measured him and he was in the healthy range for children his age: 11.5 pounds and 23.5 inches, approximately the 25th and 40th percentiles, respectively. Granted, he was taller than he was heavy, so he looked a bit thin. This disparity was a clue that something might not be going well. We measured his head circumference and it was closer to the 50 percent mark. Is Adam Lawrence representative of failure to thrive? We can't tell yet, but there are factors which suggest that something might be nutritionally amiss.

When a child is normally nourished, as a rule the height, weight, and head circumference all fall close to the same percentile curve on the growing chart. When a child becomes acutely ill or is undernourished for some reason, the weight is the first to show a decrease, followed by height, and finally by the head circumference. To some extent this is a reflection of the fact that brain growth will be preserved until the very last in the face of malnourishment. Seeing that Adam's weight is below the 25th percentile, with height around the 40th and head circumference around the 50th, we might suspect that something is amiss and that this something is possibly becoming a chronic problem, since his height is also a bit disproportionate from his head circumference. But only when Mrs. Lawrence asks the question, "Is he growing, Doctor?" do we get down to the diagnosis of failure to thrive.

Growing implies a change in height or weight over a period of time. Our suspicions that Adam may have a problem are mere speculation without evidence that there has been a change in rate of height and weight growth over the past months. For instance, it is possible that Adam was at the same percentile at birth or at two months of age as he is now. If so, we would not be concerned in the least. His growth would be seen as increasing at the appropriate rate when we take into consideration where he started from. Only if his *rate* of growth has decreased can we call him a failure-to-thrive baby. To determine whether this is the case, we must have some additional information.

"His birth weight?" Mrs. Lawrence responded to my question. "Let's see. He was a 7-pound, 2-ounce baby, and he was 20 inches long."

Both measures, on referring to the growth chart, are seen to be around the 50 percent mark. Mrs. Lawrence could not recall being told his head circumference. We now have some added information that strengthens our suspicion that Adam is failing to grow. But in the first month of life, and particularly at birth, small differences in measurements can create large differences in percentiles because the lines are clustered so closely together. Not only are we still unclear about our diagnosis of failure to thrive, but even if we were sure that Adam were indeed not growing it would be difficult to tell how long the problem had been going on. We need more information still.

"I did take him to the family doctor for his shots when he was 2 months old," she said. "Here, I have the record, and I think he also wrote in his height and weight." She handed me his immunization record.

His doctor had done a thorough job. Immunizations were recorded; height, weight, and head circumference were recorded; and an appointment had been made for two months hence. At two months of age Adam's weight looked to be near the 40 percent mark, his height was closer to the 50 percent mark, and his head circumference was also at the 50 percent mark.

"Did your doctor say anything about his growth?" I asked.

"He said he didn't think there was any problem. We talked a little about feeding techniques, and he asked me a lot of questions about how he was eating. He said we could see each other again in a month if I thought there was anything wrong; otherwise he'd see me in two months for Adam's second round of shots."

Mrs. Lawrence's doctor had done the right thing. At two months it is too early to tell if a slight variation in measurements and percentile lines is significant. He had said as much without upsetting Mrs. Lawrence and at the same time had provided a follow-up appointment to make sure the problem didn't get lost in the shuffle.

"Why did you come in to see me?" I asked out of curiosity.

"The doctor had given me your name to call if he was ever out of town—I think he's on vacation—and I was worried. I don't know. Adam just doesn't seem to be growing right."

Unless it is caused by a particularly severe problem, failure to thrive can only be diagnosed over a period of months. It takes this long to make sure the depressed growth velocity is something more than a passing phenomenon, or to make sure a temporary depression in weight isn't caused by a simple viral gastroenteritis, with vomiting and/or diarrhea, that will resolve itself in a couple of weeks. It was clear from the numbers that Adam was failing to grow. Connecting the points on his growth chart indicated that his growth curve was not as steep as those of normal children. Indirectly, this told us what we needed to know, that his growth velocity was insufficient. I say "indirectly" because the growth charts are not scaled to record actual growth velocity.

You will recall that these graphs were developed by measuring hundreds of children at every age and then joining the points together. They were not formed by taking an individual child, like Adam, and following that child's growth for eighteen years. So we can only *infer* from these curves that Adam's growth velocity is less than that of other normal children.

We have diagnosed the problem: it is failure to thrive. Now we are faced with the considerable task of determining the cause, or as doctors express it, the "etiology" of Adam's failure to thrive. Most pediatricians would agree that the major cause of failure to thrive in infancy is nutritional inadequacy, usually secondary to some feeding-associated problem in the home. The baby simply does not get enough calories to grow on. Nutritional causes, which are relatively easy to correct, need to be distinguished from other causes, which may be actual disease states—heart disease is a good example of the latter, overfeeding by the mother of the former. Identifying the possible causes of a child's failure to thrive is called establishing the "differential diagnosis."

A differential diagnosis of failure to thrive can be extremely complicated. Besides heart disease, a list of possible causes of failure to thrive might include diseases of the kidneys, thyroid, lungs, adrenal glands, pancreas, nervous system, intestines, and so on. Every organ system in the body is a potential suspect. Some causes are easier to rule out than others, but the entire testing process can be painful to the child, not to mention very time consuming and expensive. Since nutritional problems are the most common cause of failure to thrive and since they are also the easiest to correct, diagnosis should begin with this possibility.

I start by figuring out as well as I can how much the baby is eating. This means counting calories.

"How much in the past twenty-four hours?" repeated Mrs. Lawrence. "You mean, what has he eaten for breakfast, lunch, and dinner?"

"No. Actually, I want to go back to this time yesterday afternoon. Start there and tell me what you've given Adam to eat on an hourly basis."

"Well, let's see," she said. "At 4:00 P.M. he got his afternoon bottle. That was 6 ounces of formula with iron. He was hungry again at 6:00 P.M., so I gave him another. . . ."

Mrs. Lawrence went through, in detail, what is called a "twenty-four-hour dietary recall." This is one technique for assessing the adequacy of a baby's nutritional intake. It's easy to do *if* the previous twenty-four hours' feeding represents the baby's characteristic eating patterns, *if* the mother has a good memory, and *if* the baby is being bottle-fed exclusively and not breast-fed or eating solid foods. Obviously a lot of "ifs." If it becomes apparent that sufficient information won't be forthcoming via the twenty-four-hour dietary recall, I try a nutritional diary.

"How's that again?" asked Mrs. Lawrence. "You want me to write down everything I feed Adam in the next week in a loose-leaf notebook? Everything, including quantity, content, and frequency?"

"Right," I said. "To make matters easier, I want you to take these jars." I handed her two common baby-food jars of different sizes. "Write down the quantity you use of each of these jars—one-half, one-fourth, and so on—to feed Adam. Bring everything back in a week."

"That sounds like a tall order," she said.

And that's exactly the problem with *this* technique. The nutritional diary is never easy to keep.

When all else fails, I admit the baby to the hospital, where, with the help of a nutritionist, I can make a rough estimate of caloric intake per day. Hospitalization is a last resort. Hospitals are not good places for babies, or older children, for that matter. And even in-hospital diagnosis may not be easy. Still, the hospital affords the time and opportunity to watch mother and baby interact, to measure not only how much the baby takes in but also how much stays in, to weigh the baby before and after each breast-feeding to see if he is getting enough, and to weigh him on the same scales each time to see if he is growing or not growing.

The last measurement is often the most difficult to be sure about during hospitalization. A malnourished baby who is subsequently fed adequate calories may take up to two weeks to start growing again.

Once I have the baby in the hospital, I stay as close to an organized approach as I can. I allow for some flexibility, however, since clues arise when I least expect them.

The first order of business is to make sure enough calories are being provided for the baby to eat; and by enough I mean not too much as well as not too little. I try to watch the mother as she feeds her hospitalized child a formula made by the hospital or by a formula manufacturer. I watch as unobtrusively as possible, so as not to make her nervous, meanwhile talking generally about her baby's nutrition. I try to get, by the mother's account, some idea of how she prepares the baby's formula at home, since a too dilute or a too concentrated solution can lead to problems. If a mother is breast-feeding and feels uncomfortable doing so while I'm around, I ask a female nurse to observe for a couple of feedings. I weigh the baby before and after to see how much milk has been taken in.

Watching a mother feed her baby can tell me a lot. A nervous mother can make it hard for her baby to eat, since her anxiety is often transmitted to the child and can make him fret. Or the baby may be held out at arm's length and bounced continuously on the mother's knee. Dealing with anxiety can make an enormous difference, particularly when the anxiety is itself caused by maternal concern that the baby isn't eating enough. It may also be that the mother isn't the direct source of the problem. Some babies are more difficult to cuddle and console than others. A mother inevitably feels responsible for the difficult baby, and the anxiety and guilt which result may make it more difficult for her to respond to the child. The child becomes more fretful and cranky as the mother finds it more and more difficult to nurture him. I've seen remarkable changes occur in a very short time after a mother was persuaded that she shouldn't take her baby's crankiness personally.

In contrast to the nervous parent who might be underfeeding her child is the mother who is nervously overfeeding her child. Either situation can usually be discovered by the mother's account before hospitalization is necessary. On the other hand, neither may become apparent until a professional observes the child being fed. This apparent paradox—overfeeding leading to failure to grow—deserves special attention. It is not at all uncommon in this country, where we have been brought up with the idea that the only healthy baby is a chubby one. The corollary of this notion, according to some mothers I've talked to, is that a skinny baby is unhealthy and the fault of an uncaring mother.

In fact, overfeeding leading to failure to thrive turned out to be the problem with Adam Lawrence.

"Well," Mrs. Lawrence explained, "I was so worried about his not growing that I decided to give him some more to eat. I tried giving him cereals by spoon, but he didn't like them, so I added cereal to his bottle."

"What happened when you did that?" I asked.

"At first it didn't work too well, so I cut a larger hole in the nipple of the bottle and gave it to him that way. He ate so fast I thought he must be starved. So I added more and made the nipple hole a bit larger. He spit up after each feeding, but . . ."

"Are you sure he wasn't actually vomiting?" I asked.

"Well, I thought he was, but my friend said not to worry about it, that every baby spits up a little after meals. My doctor was concerned that I wasn't burping him the right way when I told him he spit up so much. Anyway, I was convinced that he wasn't getting enough to eat when he was hungry so much. He was ready to eat an hour and a half after each feeding. That was the part that made me nervous, since he seemed to be getting enough each feeding. At first I didn't want to feed him every time he cried, since I know you can spoil a baby that way, so I'd wait at least three hours in between feedings. After a while I couldn't stand his crying, so I began to feed him earlier and earlier. It made me uncomfortable, though. He was eating too often and spitting up too much."

Mrs. Lawrence was actually quite accurate in all of her perceptions. It was just that she had gotten off to the wrong start. Adam, by caloric estimate, had been getting enough to eat to begin with. By adding cereal to his bottle and cutting a larger hole in the nipple, Mrs. Lawrence was actually force-feeding him. He ate faster because he had to, with the food being delivered too rapidly through the large nipple hole. And then he vomited most of what he ate as his stomach became stretched beyond its digestive limits. Since he vomited so much with

each feeding, he was in fact being starved. Not enough calories were staying down, which is the reason he would ask for
more to eat in an unusually short time. If she had fed him
every hour and a half from the start, he might not have shown
up as a failure to thrive. He might have been obese instead—
another, but different, case of malnutrition. The fact that she
waited three hours made him voraciously hungry. He naturally ate as much as he could and as fast as he could, and then
vomited. And so the cycle went. Counting out the appropriate
amount of calories and ounces Adam was to get and giving
them to him every three to four hours solved Mrs. Lawrence's
problem.

If we determine that a child is being given the appropriate
amount of calories but he is still not growing, the problem will
probably fall into one of two areas: either he is losing too many
of the calories he is taking in, or he is using them up faster
than he can take them in.

In a sense, Mrs. Lawrence's son was losing the calories he
required for growth because he was vomiting them. His vomiting was because of a feeding problem. There are, however,
other causes of vomiting that may be more difficult to treat.
Children may vomit because of obstruction at the outlet of the
stomach, where it opens into the small intestine. This is called
"pyloric stenosis" and usually shows up in a two-week-old
child who is vomiting and not growing. In pyloric stenosis,
the vomiting is described as "projectile." It is important to
stop for a moment and consider the difference between spitting up, vomiting, and projectile vomiting.

Mrs. Lawrence was told not to worry, that "every baby spits
up a little after meals," and this is normally true. Spitting up
is when the baby brings up a little food with the burp. We
know the amount isn't significant, because a baby who is just
spitting up still grows.

Projectile vomiting is exactly what its name so graphically
suggests. It's when Daddy gets it all over his shirt and he's not
the one holding the baby. Projectile vomiting is associated with

obstruction of the outlet of the stomach (easily cured with surgery) as well as some less common and more serious diseases of the central nervous system—those associated with increased pressure inside the head. This is why it is so important to distinguish it from vomiting which is not projectile but which is of greater quantity than spitting up.

Nonprojectile vomiting may be caused by virus infections of the stomach, bacterial types of food poisonings, accidental ingestion of drugs such as aspirin or iron pills, and so on. Most of these problems are acute, though not related to failure to thrive. Still more serious diseases, such as liver failure or kidney failure, can cause a more pernicious type of vomiting. Also, psychological problems may sometimes cause persistent vomiting in older children, and these problems must be treated very seriously.

One particular type of vomiting seen in the infant that may lead to failure to thrive is called the "syndrome of infantile rumination." An unpleasant concept in its name alone, the rumination syndrome is named after the cud-chewing habit of cows and other ruminant animals, who regurgitate hastily eaten vegetable foods so that they may be rechewed and swallowed again for better digestion. The infant ruminator regurgitates his food by gagging himself, sometimes by actually sticking his little hand in his mouth. The repeated food is sometimes vomited, sometimes just spit up, and sometimes not noticed at all by the parent. In any case, the infant fails to grow. The syndrome is found most often in children who have been neglected in some way and is believed to answer their otherwise unmet oral needs. Improvement of the maternal-child bond is therapeutic in these instances.

Vomiting, then, as opposed to just spitting up, is something to be taken very seriously in a baby. I don't pretend, however, that the difference between the two is always easy to tell. And there will be the occasional time when the child who is merely spitting up will have a growth-retarding problem. The point is that growth is the determining factor. The child who is spitting up with meals but still growing at a normal rate and who is otherwise normal on physical examination does not have a serious problem.

Vomiting is one way that excessive calories can be lost. Diarrhea and other forms of abnormal or inadequate absorption of nutrients from the intestines can also cause caloric loss. Just as with vomiting, diarrhea can be caused by a number of different diseases of variable severity.

"Excuse me," said Mrs. Lawrence, slightly embarrassed. "I know this may sound silly, but could you tell me exactly what diarrhea is? I mean, by definition. The reason I ask," she added hurriedly, "is that Adam has a bowel movement sometimes three or four times a day. I told my other doctor that, but he said not to worry, that that wasn't diarrhea. I don't understand. If I went that often it would be diarrhea for sure."

"It's not a silly question at all, Mrs. Lawrence," I answered, "and it is important to make the distinction between diarrhea, which is serious, and frequent normal stools, which are not. Pediatricians are more concerned about the consistency of stools than their frequency. Diarrhea, by our definition, is a bowel movement that has too much water in it. Usually, whatever causes the increased water content also leads to an increase in the frequency of stools, which is why we adults, who have trained ourselves to have one or maybe two bowel movements each day, equate more frequent bowel movements with diarrhea. An increase in water content alters our schedule that way.

"Babies are different. As anyone who has taken care of the pre-toilet-trained child knows, babies don't have a regular schedule and can go any number of times each day. In fact, they are such anarchists that they may not even go every day, although this tendency is less common. For the most part, they have a very active gastrocolic reflex—'gastro' for stomach, and 'colic' for large intestine. An active gastrocolic reflex causes a baby to have a bowel movement after almost every time something is put in his stomach. This may mean after every meal in some normal babies, although it's usually not as active as that. Some infections of the intestines may make the gastro-colic reflex more sensitive than usual, and diarrhea is likely, particularly when every stool is mostly water. If the consistency of the stool is normal—neither too soft nor too hard—we do not have to be concerned about it. That's why your doctor was right not to get concerned about Adam's stool pattern as a cause of his failure to thrive."

"How do you know there's too much water in the stool?" Mrs. Lawrence asked. "I mean, what's the difference between the loose seedy stools that babies have when they are breast-fed and real diarrhea?"

"Water in the stool will show up as a water ring on the diaper," I answered. "A loose breast-milk stool won't have the water ring."

There are other signs of malabsorption, or poor intestinal absorption, than diarrhea as we have defined it so far. Watery diarrhea is usually the result of inflammation of the bowel wall, leading to an increased excretion of water and mucus into the stool. There are some malabsorptive states in which the intestinal wall may not be inflamed but in which enzymes necessary for the breakdown and absorption of certain food stuffs may be missing. In a disease in which these enzymes are missing, the stool may have an abnormal amount of fat in it, so it is large, bulky, foul smelling, and sort of grayish. This kind of stool is also passed with increased frequency, and the condition is called "steatorrhea." Most of the malabsorptive diseases show up with stools like this. It would be very unusual for a child who is failing to grow because of malabsorption not to display some abnormality of the stool.

Another characteristic of the child who is failing to thrive because of malabsorption is unusual appetite. Children with malabsorption frequently have voracious appetites, simply because the calories are passing right through them and not getting absorbed. As opposed to children who are starved in the presence of famine, these children are starved in the presence of plenty.

Most of the acute infections of the intestine that lead to diarrhea are of short duration and don't cause failure to thrive. We worry about them not because they lead to chronic malnutrition, but because diarrhea in an infant can cause rapid and dangerous dehydration. This is the reason, when faced with a three-month-old who probably has a viral intestinal infection, I don't worry so much about feeding the infant as I do about making sure the child gets enough fluids to replace the water that has been lost. I know the baby will be able to recover any weight lost from not taking in enough calories while ill, but may not survive if dehydration occurs. Another reason for making sure the infant takes clear fluids during acute diarrhea—and by clear fluids I mean drinks (other than plain water) that you can read a newspaper headline through (which excludes orange juice and milk)—is that during an acute diarrheal disease the moist interior lining of the intestine becomes damaged. This can affect the absorption of some normally well-absorbed sugars.

If you were to take a piece of normal intestinal wall and look at it under a microscope, you would see that the interior channel is lined with little fingerlike projections. Actually, microscopically the whole lining looks like a field of tall grass constantly in motion and is actually called the *brush border* of the intestinal wall. Every "blade of grass" contains the enzymes necessary for the digestion of various sugars. At the tip of the blade is the enzyme lactase, necessary for the digestion of lactose, the sugar found in milk.

That's what the normal intestinal lining looks like. Now suppose I take a small piece of intestinal wall from a child who had had a severe diarrhea that has lasted more than the usual three to four days—let's say a week or so. The field of grass looks like it has been cut, or even burned off in some extreme cases. No wavy motion, no tall blades; the brush border has been eroded. And the enzymes which were located here have been swept away as well. The more closely the brush border has been cut, the more different kinds of enzymes have been lost. It doesn't have to be cut much to lose lactose. If I now give this child milk with lactose in it, what will happen? The child will get more diarrhea because the lactase is not present to metabolize the lactose for absorption, and the undigested sugar in the intestine will work like a sponge to draw more water into it. This is called "transient lactase deficiency" and is a form of a potentially chronic malabsorption superimposed on an acutely malabsorptive disease. If I were not alert to the problem and kept feeding the child foods containing lactose, the diarrhea would persist, it would take longer for the intestinal lining to heal itself, and the resulting malabsorption could well lead to a failure to thrive.

"So what should a mother do?" asked Mrs. Lawrence.

"Remember first of all that this only happens after a severe diarrhea. The usual treatment for viral diarrhea is clear fluids for twenty-four to forty-eight hours, to avoid the acute malabsorption caused by the inflammation of the bowel, followed by regular formula. I usually dilute the formula half and half with water for a day or so to make it less difficult to digest, and then I go back to the original feeding schedule. It's not so difficult. The first step, clear fluids, will usually help stop the diarrhea in the first couple of days. If the diarrhea doesn't stop but rages on for days and days and boxes and boxes of diapers, you might be running the risk of a transient lactase deficiency. In this case, the regimen is clear fluids for one to two days, followed by a diluted soy formula."

"Why soy? I thought that was only for milk allergies," said Mrs. Lawrence.

"You're right. Soy formula does have a vegetable protein in it instead of a cow's milk protein, so it is used for treating allergies to cow's milk protein. But it was found that the lactose sugar in the formula was actually tied up with some leftover cow's milk protein, so the manufacturers changed the sugar as well. In most instances they have replaced the lactose with sucrose or dextrose, sugars not requiring the same enzyme as lactose for digestion. As with regular formula," I continued, "dilute the soy formula for a couple of days and then use it full strength. You may have to keep using it for two or three weeks or more."

"How will I know?"

"By trying the baby back on regular formula to see if any diarrhea develops."

"Is it true that breast-fed babies aren't susceptible to these problems?" she asked.

"It is true that they are less susceptible to bouts of infectious diarrhea, and it's also true that babies started on breast milk as early as six to twelve hours after the start of clear fluid therapy do well in most instances. They are, however, just as much at risk from the other malabsorptive diseases as other babies."

The problem of lactose malabsorption is not always the result of an intestinal infection. There are a very few reported cases of babies born with inability to digest lactose. The disease is so rare that only twenty or thirty cases of it have ever been reported. There is, however, a much higher incidence of lactose malabsorption in adults, and in some instances the problem may show up as early as two to three years of age. The inability to digest lactose, which is genetically transmitted, is found most frequently in blacks, Orientals, and native Americans. The problem is found throughout the world and results in crampy abdominal pain, diarrhea, and possibly dehydration if allowed to persist.

Another ethnically related disease causing malabsorption and failure to thrive is cystic fibrosis. Although cystic fibrosis has been detected in nearly all ethnic groups, it is found most frequently in Caucasian families of central European background, for whom the incidence is as high as 1 in 2,500 live births. As opposed to lactase deficiency, it is considerably less common (1 in 12,000 births) in American blacks.

Cystic fibrosis is another inherited disease which will show up at various ages. By one estimate, only about 50 percent of children with the disease will present in infancy. Children may present to the doctor with signs of pulmonary diseases caused by plugs of mucus in the airways, or with gastrointestinal signs of malabsorption, since the pancreas does not supply the enzymes necessary for breakdown and absorption of fats. Essentially all of the mucus-secreting glands in the body are affected by obstruction, which is the reason the pancreas cannot secrete its enzymes, the lungs are plugged with mucus, the liver shows signs of obstruction and cirrhosis, and so on. The hallmark of the disease is an increased amount of sodium and chloride in the sweat. Measurement of sweat chloride at any age is a highly reliable way of making the diagnosis.

A child who has cystic fibrosis presents with many of the signs of malabsorption we have mentioned. In the face of failure to thrive the child has a ravenous appetite, and stools are large, bulky, frequent, foul smelling, gray, and, by some descriptions, greasy.

This terrible disease is particularly important to a discussion of failure to thrive, since it provides examples of two major causes of failure to thrive: wasting calories because of malabsorption and using up too many calories because of pulmonary disease.

When children develop lung disease in cystic fibrosis, they find it more difficult to breathe because of the mucus which plugs up the small airways. When we breath in, we generate a negative pressure—a vacuum inside our chest—by expanding our rib cage and pulling down on our diaphragm. The vacuum serves to suck the air in through our nose or mouth, down our trachea, into our two large airways, through our small airways, and into our alveoli, the small air sacs where the oxygen is transferred into the blood. In the process, our small airways open to their largest diameter. On expiration, everything is reversed: the rib cage elastically recoils, the diaphragm comes up, air now loaded with carbon dioxide taken from the blood is pushed from the alveoli back up the small to the large airways, through the trachea, and out our nose or mouth. Ahhh—

we exhale. Meanwhile, our small airways have been collapsed a bit because of the pressure and because there is no longer as much air in them.

Suppose we have a mucus plug in one of the small airways. On inspiration, air will get by it as the diameter is forced open to its maximum, but on expiration we're in trouble. Air can't escape because the small airway collapses around the plug and closes off. The air that's left inside never escapes, which wouldn't be so bad except that a couple of seconds later another breath brings more air which can get in but not out. The air sac where all this air is being trapped is getting larger and larger. When we have more than one small airway obstructed in this way (as do children with cystic fibrosis or acute asthma), the chest gets larger and larger, but only a small part of it is being used for respiration. The child with this sort of lung disease has to breathe rapidly to get in more oxygen and must breathe at the top of the chest's capacity.

Try taking a deep breath, keep as much air in as you can by not exhaling as you breathe rapidly and shallowly. See how much work it takes. Imagine doing it all the time. It's not hard to understand that you would need to burn many calories just to keep breathing. When we consider that children with cystic fibrosis also have diarrhea and can't absorb the calories they do eat, it is all too apparent why they have such a dreadful rate of failure to thrive, and why before modern therapy most of them died before they were ten years old.

There are other, nonpulmonary, causes of excessive consumption of calories. Some are purely hypermetabolic—that is, metabolism is pushed to an excess—such as hyperthyroid disease or certain adrenaline-producing tumors. Chronic infections such as tuberculosis or chronic urinary tract infections fall into this category also. Some are problems of increased use of calories as well as decreased intake, like leukemia, for instance. Here the excessive energy required to produce the abnormally high number of white blood cells is frequently accompanied by a feeling of weakness, lethargy, and lack of appetite. Cyanotic heart disease is another example of such a problem: poor caloric intake because of easy fatigability in the infant is accompanied by increased metabolic demands for energy because the lack of oxygen being carried to the tissues results in anaerobic metabolism. Anaerobic metabolism, as we noted in our discussion of nutrition in athletics, is not as efficient as aerobic metabolism, so more energy must be consumed to produce the same ends, and the child consequently fails to thrive.

What happens to children who fail to thrive? If the diagnosis is made early enough to allow for nutritional supplementation, they will reverse their downward trend in growth velocity and then grow normally—assuming the problem is essentially nutritional in nature. If it is the result of a more serious disease, the prognosis may not be good. Cystic fibrosis, for example, is essentially incurable. Advances in special nutritional techniques, however, such as providing the child with all essential nutrients by vein, may help to improve the chances of failure-to-thrive victims of serious disease.

The important point is that catch-up growth can occur, and if the child's failure to thrive has been ongoing for less than a year it is not likely that brain growth, even in the sensitive months of early life, will be permanently affected. Early diagnosis is essential for a favorable prognosis.

The Crying Child

Most children who "cry too much" are not the victims of a nutritional disorder. In fact, the topic would be more suitable for a baby and child care rather than a nutritional book if it were not for the fact that, all too frequently, the bottle becomes the therapy for this common complaint. In some instances, the bottle may work, particularly in the case of a spoiled child, but this just solves one problem while creating another. In other instances, a change in diet seems to work, either because the changes in behavior that are a part of normal development occur simultaneously with the change in diet and a false cause-effect relationship is created, or because the change in diet is accompanied by an increase in attention given to the child.

An example of a misinterpreted effect of a change in diet is seen in the colicky child, who may stop crying at the age of four months regardless of diet. Another is the crying teething child, who may actually enjoy the bottle not because of its content but because of the physical rubbing of the nipple on the gums. (Teething may lead to a refusal to eat, as well, since the painful gums hurt when touched by anything.)

Crying may be perpetuated by a misinterpretation of its cause. For example, a thirsty child who is thought to be crying from hunger may be fed foods with a high renal solute load that will increase dehydration and make the infant more thirsty. Other misinterpretations may have more serious results. Infections of the middle ear (otitis media) may be painful and cause excessive crying. Gastrointestinal problems of a surgical nature which cause a sudden obstruction of the bowel may present as intermittent painful crying episodes. Increased pressure inside the baby's head, as in a serious illness such as meningitis, may make a child irritable and tearful. Other generalized infections may have the same effect. In most of these cases, however, there is evidence that something serious is going on. The onset of the crying is often more sudden. The baby looks sick, not just for a short period of time but almost constantly. And there is often an acute change in appetite and a decreased interest in food. All of this is not to say that a child who cries frequently may not be hungry, but constant crying due to inadequate caloric intake will show up, eventually, as failure to thrive. Let us consider each of the common causes of "crying too much," emphasizing the nutritional problems they may be confused with and the use or misuse of food as an antidote.

The Spoiled Child

A spoiled child is not an inherently bad child, nor are the parents of a spoiled child bad parents. The child who becomes spoiled at an early age (and most spoiled children do) has simply learned to manipulate his or her environment well enough to get his or her needs answered readily and repeatedly. As custodians of the environment, the parents of a spoiled child have allowed themselves to be manipulated in this way for a variety of reasons of their own: guilt at being bad parents, love for the child expressed as overwhelming protectiveness, or fear of what may happen if they don't respond rapidly and, as they see it, appropriately. The motives, as you see, are not appropriate for child-rearing. Parents driven by these motives find themselves more angry, frustrated, and guilty as the demands of the growing spoiled child become more and more difficult to meet. For the child, the result may be anger, impatience, and a sense of being unloved or rejected as progressively more unrealistic demands are eventually not answered.

All of these factors could be seen as distinctly non-nutritional were it not that food, used as the expression of love, as the quieter of fears ("if she eats she's all right"), or as atonement for perceived sins, inevitably enters the picture. After all, in the most simplistic terms, a baby of two months only needs three things: to sleep, to eat, to be held. The first need is in the baby's own domain, the second and the third are at the mercy of the caretaker.

So two other ills enter into our discussion of the quandary of the spoiled child, both nutritional and both with potentially far-reaching effects: the misuse of food as a reward or as an expression of love, and overfeeding with the risk of obesity.

It's difficult to say when spoiling begins. Some pediatricians believe that a baby cannot be spoiled by being picked up whenever he cries if this is done before he's three months old. Others say age makes no difference. It seems reasonable to assume, however, that a parent who responds in the first three months by picking up and feeding a baby whenever the infant cries isn't likely to change abruptly when the child becomes older than three months.

"Do you mean to say," said Mrs. Lawrence, somewhat alarmed, when she and I discussed Adam's crying habits, "that you would just leave the baby to cry, then?"

"That's not what I'm saying," I assured her. "It's always a good idea to go and find out what babies are crying about. They may need a diaper change, they may have gotten themselves in an awkward position, and they might actually be hungry. But don't forget, sometimes a baby just cries for the attention. They don't like to be neglected any more than we do. The problem with some babies is that if they had their way, they'd be commanding our attention every minute, and this mode of behavior is frequently pursued well beyond infancy. There has to be a limit. After all, the mother and father have interests of their own to pursue.

"To a large extent, establishing that limit is up to you. You're not being a bad parent if, having found out Adam is not crying about anything important, you let him cry a little. One thing I can say, however, is that food should not be used as a pacifier. Don't give him the bottle to keep him quiet. Doing that reinforces poor eating habits that will haunt you and him for years to come."

"So what should I do?" she asked.

"Give him a pacifier. Let him satisfy some of his own oral needs that way. Pacifiers are excellent for that. If crying occurs within the hour of when he usually eats, then feed him if he's hungry. But don't push it if he's not. I just don't like to see a child given a bottle every half-hour simply because he cries."

A corollary of this problem is the bedtime bottle. Getting into the habit of using a bottle to get the baby to sleep at night may cause problems, both because it fosters an attachment to the bottle as an object of security rather than as a vessel for delivering food, and because it increases the likelihood of developing serious decay of the teeth.

Problems with the Teeth

Although the subject of tooth decay and its association with nutrition is more commonly encountered in the over-one-year-old, I include it here because habits that will lead to good tooth care are developed as the teeth are erupting. In addition, dental problems hold the unique position of being both the cause and the effect of crying. The cause of crying may be teething. The effect of bedtime crying may be what we call the "nursing bottle cavity syndrome."

This syndrome is apparently the result of sugary fluid bathing the teeth all night long, leading to decay and destruction of the top front teeth. Cavities are caused by acid erosion of the tooth enamel. The acid is produced by bacteria that feed on the available sugar in the mouth. This metabolic process is called fermentation and is apparently most active in the human mouth in the presence of sucrose—common table sugar.

For the acid to be destructive to the enamel, it must be brought into close contact with it. In fact, the entire fermentation process must occur on the tooth itself for the acid to be of sufficient concentration to erode the enamel. In this instance, unfortunately, the action of cavity formation is facilitated by the interaction of the bacteria and the sugar. The product of their combination is a sticky substance called "plaque" which plasters itself against the tooth. The plaque holds the bacteria and the sugar against the tooth long enough for the fermentation process to occur and for the acid which erodes the enamel and causes the formation of the cavity to be produced.

Our body is not totally defenseless, however. If the sugar ingested is not in contact with the bacteria for a long enough time, plaque will never be formed. This is why the irrigating action of our saliva is a great preventor of cavity formation. It is, however, also why cavities form in the more poorly irrigated areas of the tooth, the fissures and crevices. Now we see why vigorous tooth brushing regularly after meals or after any sweet snack prevents cavity formation by the simple mechanical action of washing away the sugar from even the poorly irrigated areas. (Fluoride in the water or in toothpaste strengthens the enamel and makes it more resistant to erosion.)

Nursing-bottle cavities now become more understandable both in terms of why they occur and where they occur. During sleep we swallow less and we circulate less saliva in our mouth. The sugar that is in the baby's bottle—and sucrose-containing drinks are the worst but not the exclusive offenders—covers the teeth all night long. The top teeth are the affected ones since the tongue, apparently, protects the bottom teeth from the sugar content. Ample time is allowed, particularly if the bottle is given on an every-night basis, for the sugar-bacteria bond to form, causing plaque formation, fermentation, acidification, and cavitation. Before the baby who is consistently fed a bedtime bottle is two years old he'll have no front teeth, but, instead, a row of tiny blackened stumps, and maybe a painful gum abscess or two.

"I know this sounds terrible, but my neighbor brought it up and I didn't have an answer. What difference does it really make?" asked Mrs. Lawrence. "I mean really, besides cosmetic. Those are, after all, only his baby teeth. He'll get good permanent teeth to replace them, won't he?"

"The erosion of Adam's baby teeth will interfere with his ability to eat until his secondary teeth erupt, and that may not occur until he's six or seven years old. His teeth will be painful and may be the source of recurrent infections. In addition, bad care of baby teeth may lead to future problems of the same nature affecting the permanent teeth. Finally, and perhaps of greatest importance, erosion of the primary or baby teeth has a profound effect on the way that the permanent teeth come in. For appropriate positioning of a secondary tooth, it must move into a spot previously reserved by the presence of the baby tooth. If the baby tooth is no longer there, the erupting permanent tooth is displaced and may not only be unsightly but may lead to malfunction as well."

"All right. I'm convinced," said Mrs. Lawrence. "What do I do to prevent cavities in general and the nursing bottle syndrome in particular?"

"Nursing bottle cavities are easily prevented," I answered. "Stop giving the baby the bottle at bedtime."

"That's easy for you to say," she said, "but it may not be so easy to do."

"I know," I admitted. "Obviously, it's better never to get into that situation. A little foresight really is important in this case. But," I went on, "if the baby is committed to this bottle, at least take it away after he's asleep, or, better yet, give it to him with just plain water to begin with. In any case, it's bound to be a pain in the neck, which is why a pacifier or nothing at all at an early age is better than the bottle."

As for the prevention of caries, the answer is both hygienic and nutritional. Parents can start brushing their children's teeth with a soft brush when the molars are in, somewhere between a year and a year and a half. If possible, brushing after meals and snacks is best. As a child gets older, this practice becomes more and more difficult to oversee. One answer to the problem might be for parents to suggest that sweets and desserts be eaten only with meals, since brushing will be more likely after meals.

The nutritional aspect of prevention of tooth decay involves choice of foods that offer the child some sweet satisfaction with less risk of tooth decay. Fruits are superior to almost all other forms of sugar in the diet, since the fiber of the fruit helps wash the tooth as the fruit is being eaten, and the fructose sugar which is in fruits is not as likely as sucrose to cause cavities. If other sweets are eaten, the sticky, pasty kinds are most to be avoided. Their adherence to the tooth makes them act like a prepackaged plaque that just invites decay. Sweets that are delivered in a highly acidic form, as are most of the colas, can also be destructive. The acid and the sucrose provide two-thirds of the necessary ingredients for tooth decay.

The importance of fluoride from six months old on has been mentioned previously. Fluoride strengthens the enamel of the teeth. It is also important to take the child to a dentist regularly, starting when the child is two to three years old. Prevention is a key word in the dental care of the child. A healthy diet, with the right kind of sweets, along with sensible feeding habits started early in life, will do much to guarantee the future health of the baby's teeth.

"Every time the baby cries," said Mrs. Lawrence, "my mother says it's because he's teething. And this has been going on since he was four months old. She also says his teething is the cause of any fever, diarrhea—you name it. Could this possibly be true?"

"It is true that a teething child may run a low grade temperature," I answered. "And I've always heard that teething may cause some loose stools. Why, I don't know. I suspect that one of the reasons teething is blamed for so many ills is that it's almost always happening or on the verge of happening. An average child produces his first tooth sometime around seven months and continues producing baby teeth for two years. He'll start erupting his permanent teeth by the time he's six or seven years old. His last teeth may not erupt until he's a teenager."

The problem is that tooth eruption is highly variable, too variable to use as a developmental landmark. Some children have teeth visible at four months of age (an occasional child is born with a tooth), some will have none until fourteen months. As we discussed in an earlier section about fluoride and its effects, the teeth are beginning to form before the baby has been born. This is usually fairly constant. It's their appearance that may not be. The ease with which teeth appear is also quite variable. For some children it's an agonizing process—they seem perpetually cranky and fussy, maybe for weeks before the tooth erupts. For others, the tooth just seems to appear with a minimum of crankiness.

Nutrition has no effect on the teething process but may be affected by it. Some babies will not want to eat during the darker months of tooth eruption, the nipple proving too painful to their swollen gums. For them, an application to the gum of a medicine (actually the same topical anesthetic used by some dentists before they give a shot) is helpful. Applied five minutes (or less) before feeding, it will create a temporary numbing of the painful area long enough to get the bottle's contents down. The medicine is called "viscous xylocaine" and can be prescribed by any doctor. Other babies seem to enjoy the teething biscuit, the cold teething ring, or even the nipple when they are in the process of tooth eruption. In the latter instance, the calories that normally come with the nipple are beside the point—a non-nutritive nipple works just as well. The diagnosis of teething as a cause of the child's crying is necessarily dependent upon a telltale change in the appearance of the gums or the actual debut of the tooth. It's not a bad idea to put it high on your suspect list for the crying five- to six-month-old. Crying in the earlier months is less likely caused by teething and more likely the result of colic.

The Child with Colic

Colic is probably the most frustrating cause of persistent crying in the infant. It is certainly an enigmatic disorder: no one knows exactly what causes it, although many theories have been advanced, and no one knows how to treat it, let alone cure it, although many therapies have been tried. That it can have a profound and disquieting effect on a family is unquestionable. Its only saving grace is that it is apparently a self-limited disorder, usually completing its course by the time the baby is four months old.

A good part of the problem lies in the definition of the word, which derives from the same root as "colon," the large intestine. "Colic" defines a symptom and not a disease. It means "spasmodic pains in the abdomen," according to *Stedman's*

Medical Dictionary, or "a paroxysmal pain in the abdomen due to spasm, obstruction, or distention of some one of the hollow viscera," according to Webster's unabridged. As a symptom, it has no one cause, any more than fever, another symptom, has. The many causes of colic and the consequent many forms of treatment make for considerable confusion.

Colic has been described in the literature since the fifteenth century and called everything from "screaming convulsion" to "paroxysmal fussing." It has been ascribed to an immature nervous system, food allergies, problems digesting milk, and psychological stress in the child reflecting psychological tension in the family. It has even been ascribed to cold feet! Mothers who are breast-feeding are afraid colic is caused by something in their breast milk. Mothers who are bottle-feeding are convinced it occurs because they aren't breast-feeding, or they are afraid that it's something in the formula. It is one of the most common causes of multiple formula changes in infancy, certainly a more common cause than milk allergy.

It is very difficult to say what the incidence of colic is, since it is described differently in different children. For some, it may be confined to one or two bouts of acute crampy pain. The baby will let out a piercing cry, draw his legs up, his abdomen will tighten and distend, and he will turn red in the face. He really looks to be in pain. The spasm may be over in a moment, sometimes—but not invariably—after the baby passes gas. In other cases, the fussing will not be acute but persist over a variable period of time, anywhere from hours to days. During this time the baby will cry persistently, and the persistence of the crying can only be described by one who has lived through it. Some parents describe it as happening every day for one to two hours, usually between five and seven in the evening, the one time when the family is all together for dinner.

The first question parents ask after bringing their colicky child to the doctor is, "Is it dangerous?" The answer to that question is, "No, as long as we know that it's just colic and not something else." Thus, most babies are seen by a doctor during the first expression of a colicky episode. Certain diseases may present with colicky pain, and they must be excluded before the answer, "No, it's not dangerous," can be made with any assurance. The way these more serious diseases are ruled out is by examination of the baby, measurement of temperature, and occasionally examination of the stool for blood or X ray of the abdomen.

There is one childhood abdominal disease which classically presents with all the signs of colic: sudden, intermittent pain; knees drawn up; possibly passage of a diarrheal stool. It is called "intussusception" and is caused by one part of the bowel sliding over the next part—like a radio antenna being shortened. The danger of intussusception, and it is as dangerous as colic is benign, is that the blood vessels supplying that part of the bowel will get kinked and obstructed. Bowel tissue is no different from any other tissue. Without blood it will die, and what develops is an infarct of the bowel wall with passage of blood into the stool. The presence of blood in the stool is an intestinal irritant and may lead to increased action of the bowel, the result being diarrhea. Pediatricians are understandably afraid of confusing intussusception with benign infantile colic, so if the symptoms warrant, they will test the stool for blood.

After being told that their child has infantile colic and that it is not dangerous, the next question parents ask is, "How long will it last?" to which the answer is, "It's variable, but usually not more than four to six months," which immediately stimulates a final question, which is, "What do we do in the meantime?"

Some treatments for colic can be prescribed: antispasmodics for the intestines, antiflatulents for the bowel. It must be kept in mind that these are frequently mixtures of medications, which taken singly or in combination may not be the best thing for a one-month-old. It should also be mentioned that they don't always work. However, when I see family members reaching the limits of their patience, and this may happen rapidly in serious cases of infantile colic, I will prescribe medication. Usually I start at the lowest dose possible and then work my way up. But medication should be reserved for the severe cases.

Other remedies are frequently stumbled upon almost accidentally by the family. Picking the baby up and moving around with him will sometimes ease the fussing, but take note—is it colic that's made the baby cry, or is the baby spoiled and manipulating his parents? It may be very difficult to tell the difference, although the child crying for attention is more likely to stop crying if left alone for more than ten minutes. A number of parents have discovered on their way to the doctor's office that the car ride quiets the baby. They arrive somewhat chagrined with an angelic child sleeping in father's arms. The chagrin is unnecessary. The doctor is as happy as they are that the baby seems all right. (If it's the child's first bout, the doctor may still decide to check the stool for blood.) Dr. Spock suggests putting a warm hot-water bottle on the baby's tummy to relieve the spasm of the intestine. Some parents have tried feeding the baby, but whatever soothing effect occurs is usually transitory. The crying will resume in an hour or less, too soon for the baby to be hungry again. Some pediatricians say that food is the worst remedy to use since it will only intensify the spasm. Changing the formula of the colicky child has never been shown to be effective.

The point is, there is no one remedy for colic. Admitting that there is no single remedy is not meant to discount the need for particular remedies to fit particular cases. The problem in its worst expression is a serious one, which may, unless support and supervision are provided, interfere with the relationship between parents and child. It is very hard not to feel rejected by a crying child.

I am eventually left with saying to the parents of a colicky child: I understand what you are going through. I will support you through these difficult four to six months. I will try to find a treatment that will help your baby. I will supervise your attempts to do likewise. And I will make sure during these difficult months that it is always colic we are dealing with and not something more serious.

CHAPTER 10

Problems with the Toddler to the School-aged

THE TODDLER is a liberated being. Faced with choices the toddler doesn't like, he or she can become a brick wall of refusal. The most common complaint from parents of this sometimes ferociously negative individual can be summarized in these words: "I can't make him do what I want him to." The halcyon days when the individuality of this little person was more or less submerged are over. Now individuality begins to burst out all over.

Who's in Charge?

"I'm serious, doctor," said Mrs. Lawrence to me one day in Adam's second year. "I can't make him do anything I want him to. He won't eat his vegetables, he won't eat from the spoon, he doesn't like his meals when I give them to him, and he won't drink from a cup. It's awful!"

We have here a not uncommon example of a child who has taken control. When this happens, for whatever reasons, it is

[174]

difficult but necessary to remind parents that, just as in the first year, they are still the sole custodians of their child's nutritional input.

"How do I do it, then?" asked a weary Mrs. Lawrence. "How do I make him eat what I want him to eat?"

"One thing to remember," I reminded her, "is that no one likes to be forced to do anything. As often as possible, let Adam exercise his independence and individuality by choosing from alternatives and by giving him some control over his own intake. Let him feed himself the finger foods, let him use the cup, let him try out his talents on the spoon. Children are great imitators. Left to their own devices they will become, sometimes embarrassingly, like us."

"Choices?"

"This vegetable, or that vegetable, or . . ."

"But what if he won't take either?" she interrupted.

"That's the third choice—or nothing that meal. Remember that a balanced diet is balanced per week, not per meal. There will come a meal that is heavy on vegetables. If he really doesn't want to eat them, he doesn't have to. Don't argue or coax. It's his choice. Then, business as usual next meal. He'll undoubtedly be hungrier the next time around and will probably find that vegetables are just fine."

"I hate to see him hungry."

"You also hate to see him not eating the foods you know are good for him. Once he knows he can outlast you and get milk or whatever else he wants instead, things become more difficult. And once he's older and can feed himself, things can become impossible. You're not punishing him for not eating—he's just learning about choices."

"Should I give him vitamins to stimulate his appetite?" she asked.

"Vitamins really don't stimulate appetite. Vitamins should be used to supplement the diets of severely malnourished children, children with intestinal malabsorption, or children who are too debilitated to eat a regular diet. Remember, after a year he doesn't have as big an appetite as before. His growth rate has decreased, and so have his requirements for calories. Don't force-feed him."

"But don't you think he looks skinny?" she asked.

"He doesn't look fat," I said. "He's growing just above the 40 percent mark for his height and the 35 percent mark for his weight, according to the growth chart. He's growing at the appropriate rate for both. That's healthy. He doesn't need to be chubby to be healthy, despite what our society says. Skinny? You may call him skinny, but it's okay if he's skinny. He'll probably stay skinny all his life, which may end up being longer as a result. Let's spend some time talking about being too fat. Let's discuss obesity. We'll discuss it from all perspectives: how it is defined, the various theories of what causes it, what problems it's associated with, and how to treat it. It may seem strange to discuss it when Adam is this age, and skinny as well, but preventing obesity is all too clearly superior to treating it. You can never start too soon."

Obesity

Any discussion of obesity must begin with a clear definition of the word, since the meaning changes with almost every individual who uses it. In some cases it reflects an overestimation of a problem: the teenager who is 6 to 10 pounds overweight says "I'm obese" and goes on a crash diet. In other cases, the problem is underestimated: the little six-month-old with the extra chins who can't bring his legs together isn't called "obese," he's called "chubby."

It's one thing to say of oneself, in a self-deprecating sort of way, "I really should not eat so much, I'm getting obese." It's quite another thing if someone else agrees. No one takes being called obese as a compliment. Obesity bears a distinct stigma. Try as they might to view the obese sympathetically, as individuals unable to control a disorder that has possibly afflicted them since childhood, the non-obese often feel a sense of self-righteous disgust in the presence of the obese. "How can *any-one* let themselves get into that condition—absolutely no self-control." The not-so-subtle implication is that if the obese led a good clean life—"like I do, which is why I'm not obese; maybe a few pounds over, but not obese"—they too would reap the benefits of a low-calorie life, under the benevolent gaze of a lean God.

So, in an effort to remove the stigma which surrounds obesity, and in recognition of the fact that emotionally derived definitions are inexact, we will try to define obesity in more medical terms. I say "try" because we aren't out of the woods yet. The medical/nutritional community has had almost as much difficulty defining obesity as it has had measuring it. In fact, the two are virtually inseparable.

Turning once again to *Stedman's Medical Dictionary*, we find "obesity: an abnormal increase of fat in the subcutaneous tissue." This definition is not terribly useful either for research or for practice. What is meant by "abnormal"? The Oxford English Dictionary is of little more help: "obesity: excessive fatness or corpulence." However, it does tell us that "obesity" comes from the Latin *"obesus:* that which has eaten itself fat, stout, plump." We gather from this that obesity is associated with the fat component of the body that is increased through eating. This quality at least distinguishes it from the concept of overweight. A weight-lifter may be overweight for his height and body type, because lean body mass weighs more than fat does, but you wouldn't call him (or her) obese—at least not to his face.

So how do we measure the fat component—called the "adipose tissue"—of the body as distinct from the other components of weight: bones, water, blood volume, and muscle? In a research setting we could go to considerable lengths. We could measure the body's water and blood volume, add the weight of that to the weight of lean body mass, which is estimated by measuring the total body potassium, found largely in muscle cells, and subtract that sum from the total body weight. The difference would be a close estimate of the weight of adipose tissue. Or, because fat has greater mass than muscle and therefore displaces more water, we could employ the principle of Archimedes and submerge someone in a vat of water and measure how much water volume is displaced. Accurate, but not ideal for the obese cardiac patient, and certainly not suitable for the doctor's office.

Let's go back to the dictionary definition that read, "an abnormal increase of fat in the subcutaneous tissue." "Subcutaneous" at least tells us what to look at—at the tissue under the skin. That's what researchers have done in developing a method of measuring "skinfold thickness" or, as it has been more recently termed, "fatfold thickness."

The measurement of skinfold is done by pinching the back of the arm (tricep skinfold) or the tissue under the shoulder blade (scapular skinfold), holding it out for a short but specific time, and measuring its thickness with a finely calibrated caliper. What we are measuring is two thicknesses of skin and the tissue underneath. Skin thickness is relatively constant from one individual to another and certainly doesn't vary with fatness the way the subcutaneous tissue does. The tissue underneath is the adipose tissue we are looking for. By comparing a large number of these measurements on a wide variety of people who are thin, average, or fat, we come up with a range of variability similar to that of the growth chart. There is an upper limit to what would be considered normal in skinfold thickness, and anyone who is above that limit can be considered obese.

Although measurement of skinfold thickness is not quite accurate enough for use in most medical research, it has found increasing use in the office as more and more practitioners familiarize themselves with the technique and invest in the somewhat expensive calipers needed for the assay. (We've come a long way from grandmother's pinch on the cheek. She was, however, performing a skinfold thickness test at considerably less expense.)

The introduction of skinfold measurements is quite recent, owing in large part to the absence of standards with which they could be compared. It has been only in the past few years that enough measurements have been made on enough children of all ages to give us the range of what may be considered normal.

In the absence of this more recent test, obesity continues to be measured by more traditional means—once again, not really accurate enough for research but suitable for practice. The age-old measure is the comparison of weight and height. In this technique, after plotting the child's height and weight on the usual growth charts, another graph is used to compare his weight with his height. If Jimmy Jones' weight is at the 75th percentile for his age and his height is at the 30th percentile, Jimmy is heavier than he is tall. How much heavier? Well, on his weight-compared-to-height graph he is at the 95th percentile. A child whose weight is appropriate for his height will be at the 50th percentile. The 95th percentile means Jimmy Jones' weight-to-height ratio is greater than the weight/height ratio of 95 percent of other children. (Weight-to-height graphs are reproduced on pages 233–236.) This means he is significantly heavier than he should be at his height.

The problem with this form of definition is that it equates weight with obesity. Some kids with massive skeletal frames might have an elevated weight-to-height ratio even if they aren't obese. At this point we have to return once again to dear old grandmother. We measure a child's weight-to-height ratio at a given age, and then we look at him. Obese children look like obese babies. Grandma knew, only obesity was frequently a sign of health to her generation. You can *see* the subcutaneous fat on the obese child. On obese children or babies there are extra skinfolds, extra chins, and extra tissue in general. Most children are not weight-lifters. If their weight-to-height ratio is over the 95 percent mark, they are obese.

Now that we have a working definition of obesity and have formulated some ways to measure it, we can see that we are dealing with a problem that is on a different scale from that of the adolescent who is 10 pounds overweight. The definition must be made by looking at the proportion of weight and height. Ten pounds in a 120-pound adolescent is insignificant. However, Jimmy Jones, who was obese by our definition, only had to lose 4 pounds to attain ideal weight for his height. When we discuss cause and effect of obesity, we want to be sure we are studying the truly obese.

The cause of obesity is deceptively simple: more calories are consumed than are used up. We term this explanation deceptively simple because it tells us nothing about why more calories are consumed or why fewer calories are used up. It tells us nothing about the cases that seem to contradict this simple formulation of the cause of obesity. Some obese individuals exercise but are still obese; some consume a diet of average caloric intake but maintain their obesity.

The further one probes into the cause of obesity, the more complex and confusing it becomes. The theories developed to explain obesity are as plentiful as those developed to explain colic. It is becoming ever more apparent that obesity is the end expression of many disorders.

"I don't understand," said Mrs. Lawrence. "Once people decide that they are obese and that they don't want to be so any longer, they go on a diet to lose the pounds and maybe exercise more. Why all this concern about cause when the solution to the problem is the same, regardless of cause?"

"That's a valid point," I said. "But for those who are obese enough to want to lose weight, the success rate is pretty grim. Of the obese individuals who go on reducing diets and lose to their ideal weight, only 5 *percent* will remain at that ideal weight over the next five years. Those aren't very good odds. That's the reason more and more people are investigating the causes of obesity with an eye to preventing it, since treating it has proven to be so unsuccessful. It is also the reason obesity has become a pediatric topic, since the prevention of obesity begins in childhood, maybe even in the first six months of life."

"So if you're already obese you shouldn't even bother trying to diet, from the sound of things," said Mrs. Lawrence.

"Well, I know it sounds discouraging, but that's not really the point. At the same time people have been investigating the causes of obesity, others have been looking into better ways to diet. We'll talk about those as well," I told her. "But let's go back to the causes of obesity.

"When I was in grade school, I remember, one of my classmates was very obese. Interestingly, she was not only obese but tall as well, just not tall enough. Her weight-to-height ratio was still abnormal. Because she was so obese, everyone said that she must have a glandular problem, meaning she had some sort of hormonal imbalance. I mention this case first because this perception of obesity is as common now as it was then. It is usually inaccurate. In fact, 'glandular' problems—hormonal imbalances caused by abnormalities of the thyroid gland, the adrenal gland, or the structures of the brain that stimulate these glandular organs—are *extremely* rare causes of obesity. This is not to say they never occur. There are theories which point in particular to abnormalities of that area in the brain, the hypothalamus, that governs the actions of these glands. The hypothalamus is instrumental in giving us our sensation of hunger and satiety."

Appetite is different from hunger. Our appetite originates from areas in the brain apart from the hypothalamus and involves certain psychological elements, including the pleasurable anticipation of food, that are probably independent of the nutritional value of food. Appetite can be affected by psychological associations, like looking forward to a meal because it represents a safe time with the family devoid of stress. It is highly possible that appetite abnormalities, which control hunger and satiation, may be the cause of many cases of obesity.

Two parts of the hypothalamus are known to affect hunger

and appetite: a medial part closer to the center of the brain and a lateral part closer to the brain's surface. The medial part houses what is known as the "satiety center." It is hardly as exciting as its name suggests. A "satiety center" should be somewhere you could go to have all your desires granted. Actually, our inner satiety center controls our desire to eat. When the satiety center is stimulated, we perceive fullness and stop eating; were it removed or malfunctional, we would be inclined to indulge ourselves in food. Exactly how it is stimulated is another question. Possibly nerves from the stomach that perceive the stretching following a meal send out messages to the hypothalamus which stimulate it; possibly it is stimulated by the level of glucose, insulin, or fat in the blood following a meal; or possibly it is stimulated by the lateral part of the hypothalamus. The lateral part of the hypothalamus is called the "hunger center." Stimulation of this area excites hunger; removal of it would remove our perception of hunger.

The medial and lateral areas are obviously essential for normal eating patterns, and their interaction is a finely balanced one. Researchers theorize that an imbalance between the two, e.g., hunger being dominant over satiety, may be a cause of obesity. This may be so, but it raises other questions: why the imbalance? what causes it? Indirect support for this theory of hypothalamic imbalance as a cause of obesity was provided by a study of the victims of a famine during World War II when the inhabitants of the northwestern part of the Netherlands were being besieged by the Nazis, who strictly limited the food imported to that area. The result was six months of famine— the average caloric intake fell to between 800 and 900 calories per person per day. Research done twenty years later showed that babies of mothers subjected to the famine during the first two trimesters of pregnancy had an increased rate of obesity later in life compared to babies of mothers who were well fed. Babies who were starved in the last trimester and immediately after birth had a decreased incidence of obesity. One of the theories advanced to explain this discrepancy is that because the hypothalamus is in the developmental stage during the first two trimesters, babies who had been starved at this stage of their fetal development tended toward malfunction of the hypothalamus in later life.

It has also been theorized that hypothalamic malfunction and some other factors which lead to obesity are passed on genetically from parent to child. This theory is bolstered by the well-known fact that a child with one obese parent has a much greater likelihood of being obese by the time he is seven years old than a child with two lean parents. Having both parents who are obese increases the likelihood of being obese later in life even more. One major argument against this theory arises from the difficulty in sorting out the inherited effects from the environmental. Certainly, if one or more parent is obese (and it doesn't make any difference which parent), the chances are that overeating is encouraged within the family. Perhaps food is even regarded as a reward for good behavior. In an effort to resolve the genetic versus environmental problem, researchers in Scandinavia looked at twins who had been separated at birth and brought up in different homes. They found that although the twins were slightly different in weight, they were still closer to each other in this regard than the children of their adoptive parents. Genetic studies have shed light on a possible factor in obesity but have not provided the complete answer. There are, after all, children of obese parents who are not obese and children of lean parents who are. In the final analysis, the effect of the home environment cannot be totally discounted.

For those who believe that the tendency toward obesity is acquired after birth and not totally inherited, the question is how early in life it is acquired. The answer: it can be acquired very soon after birth. It is known that infants who grow rapidly in the first six months of life are more prone to obesity later on. The cause for this may be related to the number of fat cells created during that time. Researchers in this country have shown that obesity that begins in adult life is associated with an increase in the size of the fat cells alone, whereas obesity that begins in childhood is associated not only with large fat cells but also with an increased number of them. It is easier to reduce the size of the fat cell by dieting than to reduce the number of them. The investigators who discovered this association suggest that there are times in life when the body is more prone to make more cells. Those periods roughly coincide with the rapid growth spurts in the first six months of life and during adolescence. This is a pragmatically promising theory of obesity in that it indicates two periods of time when obesity might be targeted for prevention. It corresponds to information gained from a separate and independent study that showed that children whose weight was above the 75 percent mark on the growth chart by six months of age had a greater risk of developing obesity before seven years of age than children whose weight remained below that percentile. If it is, in fact, true that the first six months of life are critical to the onset of obesity, it becomes very important indeed that we not overfeed the baby with calorie-concentrated solid foods during these months.

All of these theories implicate too much intake as the major cause of obesity. Skeptics of these theories are quick to point out that some obese individuals do not ingest an abnormally great amount of calories each day, but actually eat less than other individuals who never become obese. They contend that intake of calories cannot be the only answer. Perhaps a decrease in expenditure of calories through decreased activity or a reduction in requirements for energy to maintain body heat is at the root of such cases.

If one watches obese children playing games with non-obese children, it is evident that the obese are less active than the non-obese. But which came first, obesity or loss of activity? Have these children become obese because they are less active, or are they less active because they are obese? After all, carrying around a sizable number of extra pounds can do a lot to limit your interest in moving around fast. One recent study of a small number of children at play showed that although obese children were somewhat less active than their non-obese peers, their weight problem still lay in their overconsumption of calories.

Other investigators have studied the thermogenetic, or heat producing, capability of obese children, testing the theory that the increased fat layer on the bodies of these children leads to less requirement for heat production to maintain normal body temperature. Obese children are, in effect, better insulated, but this does not explain how they got to be obese in the first place. Perhaps they had abnormal mechanisms for heat production to begin with. For example, after a large meal the body tends to increase its heat production so that extra calories taken in will be burned up rather than stored as fat. The tissue that allows this increase in heat production is called "brown fat," a particular kind of fat unlike the white fat responsible for insulation and the appearance of fatness. Brown fat is located in various parts of the body—around the major blood vessels deep in the chest, around the kidneys, and in the area of the back between the two scapulas. Brown fat is also responsible for the cold-induced increase in body heat that is the body's nonshivering response to a drop in the environmental temperature. When "turned on" by a meal or by the cold, the brown fat starts burning up calories and producing heat. Recent studies suggest that the brown fat mechanism in the obese may not work as well as it does in the non-obese. In those with malfunctioning brown fat, extra calories will not be burned up in heat production but stored as white fat instead.

This variability in function may explain why some people can apparently indulge themselves with impunity and never become obese, whereas others who indulge themselves to the same extent rapidly and inexorably become fat. Brown fat studies are inconclusive but encouraging. So far, however, no practical treatment for obesity has emerged from them.

We turn now to causes of obesity which have more to do with appetite and psychologically related phenomena than with metabolically induced increases in intake or decreases in output. They have to do with the development of eating habits and use of food. We know that people with a tendency toward being obese will respond to stress or depression by eating more, whereas people who tend to be lean respond to the same stimuli by eating less. How these behavioral differences have developed is unknown. A mother of one of my patients insists the tendency to overeat under stress develops because food is used as a reward. Although not obese herself, she has found herself tending toward being overweight. She recognizes her tendency to go to the refrigerator whenever she is feeling down in the dumps. Although she never uses food to reward her children, when her mother comes over she witnesses an all too familiar scene from her own childhood: "If you eat your peas, I'll give you ice cream for dessert." Does a person become obese because food was used as a reward in childhood, or because the only way he or she received any nurturing was by self-nurturing with food? In any case, if food has become an overweeningly important psychological stimulus in a person's life, one must be very careful that removing the stimulus does not result in more serious psychological harm. This type of situation reflects the complexity of the obesity problem and underscores how important prevention of that problem is.

"If we don't know exactly what causes obesity," said Mrs. Lawrence, "how can I possibly prevent Adam from becoming obese?"

"Well," I said, "let's consider some of the common features of the various theories about obesity.

"We have to concentrate on the first months and years of life, since enough studies have indicated that fat infants are more likely to be fat adults. First, breast-feeding probably leads to less obesity, not because a baby cannot become obese on breast milk—he can—but because breast-fed babies tend to start solid foods later in life than bottle-fed babies do. Second, the early introduction of solid foods predisposes to overeating and obesity for a number of reasons: the increased intake of concentrated calories which the baby has no control over, the increased renal solute load leading to thirst that may be misinterpreted by baby and parent as increased hunger, and the tendency of some parents to answer all the baby's need for attention with food. Third, a baby should be fed when he's hungry and at no other time. This is important not only during infancy but during the second and third years of life as well. Remember that these are the years during which you, the parent, have the greatest control over what the child eats and how the child eats. If we refuse to allow ourselves to be manipulated by the stubborn ways, or even the charming ways, of our one-to-two-year-olds, we will be doing them a great favor. You understand what is necessary for a normal and well-balanced diet. Constantly giving in to a child's preference for sweets or other high-calorie food is no sign of love in the long run.

"For prevention to work it must be started in the early months and years. By the time children are in school or become adolescents, they have their own means of dealing with their appetites—notice I didn't say hunger. We hope by that age they will have become habituated to the use of healthful foods as a healthful response to hunger."

Problems Associated with Obesity

"Tell me something," said Mrs. Lawrence. "I know that being obese as an adult is associated with heart disease, high blood pressure, and diabetes. Obese people aren't supposed to live as long. But let's say that my child grows up with immense willpower, so that although he may be fat through his adolescence, by the time he's in college he decides to lose weight—and he does it, and not only that, but he's one of the 5 percent who stay at their ideal weight. If that were to be the case, what difference would it make if he were fat as a child?"

"First of all, that would be an awful lot of willpower, but I'll grant you it is definitely possible. What goes against it is the fact that the patterns which we develop as children are hard to break as adults, but again by no means impossible, and I have known children who grew up to do exactly what you described. To answer your question, there are few medical problems in childhood related to obesity. Most obesity-related problems are orthopedic and stem from excess strain placed on the joints by the child's weight. But there are also psychological problems. Fat kids have a hard time with their peers because they are distinctly different, and they know it. The girl in my grade-school class whom I mentioned before was an outcast. She got chosen last for games, she was called unkind names, and no one wanted to sit next to her in class. Her life, I now see in retrospect, must have been miserable."

"At what age are fat children aware of their obesity?" asked Mrs. Lawrence.

"It used to be thought that the only kids who felt ostracized by their obesity were adolescents. And that was because they didn't get asked out on dates. But the social sanctions against the obese don't start or stop there. Studies have shown that obese people have a harder time getting into college and getting jobs. It's a shame when you realize that obesity is a problem which is most likely not of their own making. When you ask obese adolescents to tell you when they first thought they were too fat, most of them will tell you it was around seven or eight years old. This is an interesting age in the child's cognitive development. It is an age when children come outside themselves, when they begin to see themselves as others see them. They no longer see the whole world from the ego's point of view. It's an absolutely appropriate age for a child to notice that others are treating him differently and to become aware of why this is so.

"The reactions of obese children to their 'differentness' can be very poignant. When I asked one nine-year-old girl why she wanted to lose weight, she said, 'Because I'll be healthier and live longer.' We talked at greater length. She admitted she really wasn't sure how it would make her healthier—she felt pretty good and could ride her bicycle as well as any kid on the block. She also wasn't sure what it meant to live longer. I questioned her gently but more firmly. Finally she admitted, tears streaming, that it was really because of all the names the other kids called her and that she was afraid to go away to summer camp.

"This humiliation is the major problem of obesity in childhood as I see it. It may be argued that psychotherapy is more important for the child than nutritional therapy, but I believe it is asking too much to tell a child to feel good about himself or herself no matter what other kids think or say. The old 'sticks and stones will break my bones, but names will never hurt me' adage is just not true. Names do hurt. The effect on a child's later development may be profound, and for this, if for no other reason, one should work very hard to prevent childhood obesity."

"As a parent," Mrs. Lawrence asked, "what can I do if my child is seven or eight years old and obese? Let's say Adam doesn't lose whatever extra weight he has on his bones when he's very young—what do I do later?"

"The first and cardinal rule for weight reduction in the growing child—and we'll consider the treatment from a developmental point of view—is to remember that your primary concern is not to make the child lose weight. I know this sounds contradictory. But weight reduction as an all-encompassing goal can lead to diets which might be very dangerous for the growth and maturation of various organ systems that are in special need of normal calories. Think of it this way: you will be letting the child's height catch up to his weight. That's the best rule of thumb I know.

"For instance," I continued, "Mrs. Smith is concerned that her four-month-old son John is too fat, or is going to grow up like his father, who certainly is. She puts her son on a skim milk diet. Johnny may eat fewer calories—skim milk has half the calories of whole milk—but now 100 percent of his calories are made up of carbohydrates and protein, more than his kidneys can manage when it comes to renal solute load. Johnny loses weight, but he may lose too much, and his diet has become too unbalanced. He gets no essential fatty acids, he gets no cholesterol, and he may not get enough calories for normal growth of his brain and his height.

"The same is true at any age in a growing and developing child. The crash diet and the starvation diet have no place in pediatrics. Reduction in weight should come by way of a balanced reduction of caloric intake. What this usually means is feeding an obese child the calories at the lower limit of what is necessary for growth in height and head circumference. For instance, a one-year-old needs anywhere from 40 to 50 calories per pound of body weight per day for normal growth. If the child has been growing at too rapid a rate, sit down with your pediatrician and calculate the number of calories he is getting. It will probably exceed the 50-calories-per-pound mark. Devise a balanced reduction and start feeding him 35 calories per pound per day. In the meantime, follow his growth chart—in this case his height-for-age growth—and make sure he continues growing along the appropriate curve. If his height is increasing and his weight also continues to increase, reduce the calories a bit more.

"In the preschooler, weight gain is most frequently tied up with too many calories being eaten, but don't neglect the exercise side of the equation. Encouraging your child to exercise when he becomes restless or fidgety serves two purposes: it burns up calories and removes your temptation to feed him in order to quiet him down.

"It is useful to remember that dieting for the grade-school age child may require a change in the eating habits of the entire family, especially when one or both parents are obese. But it may also be necessary when both parents are lean. When a child has grown up enough to have access to the refrigerator, the only way to make sure that the food he gets at home is nutritious and not particularly fattening is to have only nutritious and nonfattening food at home. This may mean that a lot of the foods which are family favorites will have to go. It may also mean that mom and dad and brother and sister will end up eating fruit and carrot sticks after school and before bed, instead of cookies and chocolate milk. In anticipation of such problems and possible tensions, I try to meet with the entire family, or at least the parents, at the outset of treatment of an obese child."

"What if they want their child admitted to the hospital for weight reduction?" asked Mrs. Lawrence.

"That is occasionally necessary, particularly for the very obese. But I try to avoid it whenever possible."

"How come? Because it's so traumatic to the child to be put in the hospital?"

"Well, there's that reason. And others. First of all, when you admit a child to the hospital, you are telling that child and the rest of the family that this is the child's problem, and there may even be the implication that it's the child's fault. This is unfair. Being obese can hardly be considered an eight-year-old's fault. The problem began long before, and its causes probably center in the home. That brings up another reason I try to avoid hospitalization. The child gets admitted to the hospital. The child loses weight because we've provided him or her with an absolutely controlled dietary environment. The child has no choice in the matter. What do you suppose will happen as soon as the child returns home to the same temptations and to the same familial patterns that led to obesity to begin with?"

"But doesn't it give the child a headstart, let him realize how good he feels once he's lost the weight?"

"And won't he feel especially depressed," I answered, "when there is no support at home to help him maintain his ideal weight? The pounds, I can assure you, will reappear."

"How about if you were to work with the family while the child was in the hospital?" she asked.

"That's a good idea, a very good idea, since it helps shift the blame away from the child. And that's actually what I try to do in the particularly recalcitrant cases. But the hospitalized child still bears the stigma of being 'afflicted.' In addition, hospital treatment may isolate the patient to an extent that it prevents the family from gaining true insight into their role in the problem."

"All right," she said, "I'm convinced."

Another very important point I emphasize to the obese child and the child's family is that the reduction in weight may be painstakingly slow. Some adults who are *starved* lose only about one pound a day, and children who are on calorie-restricted diets may lose only a half-pound a day or less, depending on the restriction. The rapidity with which a negative calorie balance may be reached—that is, more calories being used up than taken in—can be accelerated by exercise as well. Exercise alone, however, will not work. In fact, many individuals use exercise as an excuse to eat more. Exercise is beneficial in a variety of ways: it increases caloric expenditure; it can serve as a positive substitute for negative behavior (i.e., overeating); and it is good for overall health and well-being. In many instances, entire families have become involved in a healthful exercise program in order to help their child break habits that have led to obesity—too much television, perhaps, or too much time spent within easy reach of the refrigerator.

Treatment of obesity in the school-age child often involves altering mealtime behavior. It has been shown that many obese children tend to eat very quickly. In fact, one of the theories for their obesity is that they eat so fast that the normal mechanisms which sense appetite fulfillment do not have time to be activated before an excessive amount of calories has been eaten. In order to thwart this cycle of events, therapists interested in the modification of behavior have come up with a number of recommendations. They suggest, for example, that parents make sure the child puts his or her fork down between each mouthful until it is swallowed. They also recommend a three- to five-minute break in the middle of each meal to allow the family to talk, socialize, and thus gain more time for the body's appetite suppressant mechanisms to come into play. And they suggest that smaller portions be placed on the plate so that even if the child should fail to slow down, the total number of calories eaten will still be reduced. These techniques and others like them accentuate once again the importance of family participation in treatment of the obese child.

Diets themselves, the types you or I or our adolescent children might go on, are discussed in detail in the next chapter. The ideal diet has two components: weight reduction and weight maintenance. The weight reduction diet taxes the child and the family, but the difficulties are relatively short lived. They end when the weight considered appropriate for the child is reached. Weight maintenance diets, on the other hand, are essentially life-long efforts.

The Effects of Nutrition on Behavior

"It would be fascinating to read a book on how nutrition affects behavior," a friend of mine recently remarked.

I agreed but pointed out that it would be a very short book indeed, since very little is really known about the effects of nutrition on behavior.

"Oh, go on," he said. "All this business about additives and hyperactivity, megavitamins for all kinds of behavior problems, the evils of table sugar. One could certainly write a book about that."

"Some have," I said, "but the 'data' they use are very sketchy and consist mostly of anecdotes from their own experience. I'm not saying personal observations are not important—they're the source of many scientific breakthroughs—but to become more than a source for further speculation they have to be tested. It's in the testing that most of these 'data' shatter. Some speculations about nutrition's effect on behavior are total mythology—like eating a lot of fish because it's 'brain food.' Fish is no more brain food than any other food. Other misconceptions are based on accurate observations but inaccurate conclusions—for instance, feeding a child protein before he's sent to school so that he'll be more attentive during class. We know children need breakfast in the morning, but as a source of carbohydrates that keep the blood sugar up until lunchtime. Protein won't have an effect on them during the morning. Protein isn't a quick energy source. It takes longer than a few hours for it to be absorbed from the gastrointestinal tract and incorporated into enzyme and cellular constructions. We do know that if children eat the wrong kind of carbohydrates exclusively, simple carbohydrates like sucrose instead of complex carbohydrates like starches, the subsequent leap in insulin levels will bring the sugar level down too fast and may make them irritable by late morning."

"But there, you said sugars alter behavior. There's an example," my friend persisted.

"Yes, but I'm not suggesting all sucrose be removed from the diet, I'm simply asking that the diet be maintained in balance. The same is true when you talk about vitamins. Sure, they're important—we couldn't live without them. But they're appropriately called micronutrients because we only need small amounts of them to live and grow normally. When vitamins are given in megadoses they are no longer micronutrients, they have become hardly different from new medications, the unwanted effects of which have yet to be completely revealed. Some of them, like vitamin A or vitamin D, are known to be toxic . . ."

"Toxic?"

"Poisonous if taken in large doses for prolonged periods of time. That's because they're stored in the body fat and not readily excreted. Others, like vitamin C, are not stored but are readily excreted in the urine. When taken in excessive amounts, a good part of vitamin C ends up in the toilet."

"And I remember you telling me once that megadoses of vitamin C have not been proved to be helpful in preventing colds."

"That's right. Now, it is possible that people who take megavitamins when they do have a cold feel better, but there's no proof it's because of the vitamins. They may feel better simply because they're doing something *they think* will help them. Children whose parents give them high-dose vitamins may even get fewer colds, but that could be because of the increased attention they are getting and the fact that other precautions are being taken to keep them well. If they have a cold and take vitamin C, they may feel better simply because they are taking in a lot of fluids with the vitamin C. I am not trying to diminish the importance of trying to take good care of yourself or your children. But it bothers me that many people feel they must take pills to accomplish this.

"It also bothers me when food is viewed as a medication or as the cause of a child's behavioral problem. Imagine how you would feel about food in general if you thought that what you ate was making you do bad things."

"Hey! What a great alibi that would be."

"It might be. But if the truth of the matter is that food is not the cause of your bad behavior or your child's, you could spend a lot of time pursuing answers to the wrong questions if you were a research nutritionist or a concerned parent. To a large extent, I think that's what has happened with our study of hyperactivity in children, especially in terms of food additives causing hyperactivity."

"Didn't hyperactivity once have another name?" asked my friend.

"Yes. It used to be called 'minimal brain dysfunction,' but then, because a number of pediatricians and pediatric neurologists argued that there was no proof it had anything to do with brain dysfunction at all, it was changed to 'attention deficit disorder,' the major symptom of which is hyperkinesis—another term for hyperactivity.

"In 1973 Dr. Ben Feingold, a pediatrician interested in child allergies, made some observations that led him to believe that naturally occurring compounds called salicylates, which are very closely related chemically to aspirin, might be responsible for hyperactivity. Dr. Feingold had noted that children with aspirin intolerance showed many of the same symptoms of hyperactivity as kids with attention deficit disorders."

"What exactly *is* hyperactivity?" my friend asked. "I mean, I don't want to appear stupid, but aren't an awful lot of normal grade-school kids pretty active?"

"That's by no means a stupid observation. Part of the problem in studying the effects of either medicine or diet on hyperactivity has been that it is so difficult to define. Essentially you're correct: many normal children are constantly on the move. They've got incredible energy levels. They move around a lot, seem restless, and get into everything. But when something engrosses them, when some task or toy captures their interest, they attend to it and may stay engrossed in it for hours. Not so the hyperkinetic child. He is usually easily picked out in the office waiting room—otherwise the office would probably be destroyed. He is so active, particularly in the stressful condition of a doctor's office, that he never stops moving around—nothing holds his attention for long. He sees something he likes, holds it, looks it over, seems about to play with it—then something else catches his eye and he's off to the new stimulus. He seems literally driven. He may present with a sleep problem or intense anxiety. Or he may even show failure to thrive because he is not able to sit still long enough to concentrate on eating."

"What can be done about hyperactivity? Is there no treatment at all?" my friend asked.

"There are treatments. Some of them are medicinal. You give the child methylphenidate or dexamethasone, two drugs which speed up activity in normal children but have the opposite effect on children with hyperkinetic disorders. I have used these drugs, but very rarely and only in extreme cases. I remember using methylphenidate with one extremely hyperkinetic patient of mine until I visited his home and witnessed what was happening in the home environment. The child was trying to do anything he could to please his parents and gain their attention. They were ignoring him, and the more they did, the more hyperactive he became. I stopped the pills. The problem was more psychological than physiological. In another case, a child labeled hyperactive at school was sent to me for medication, but it didn't seem necessary. He actually sat quietly in my office. But when he tried to do the psychological test we presented to him, he couldn't sit still. As it turned out, he had a language problem, and no matter how hard he tried, he couldn't keep up with his schoolwork. After a while, he stopped trying. He spent his school time in pointless activity and disruptive behavior. All he wanted to do was get out of class and away from its threatening environment."

"That's very interesting," commented my friend. "But where does Dr. Feingold fit into all this?"

I went on to explain that Feingold extended his original theory that salicylates in food caused hyperactivity. He put food preservatives under the same indictment. Since preservatives are so widely used, Feingold's final list of forbidden fruits is extensive and includes many fruits and vegetables, tea, coffee, margarine and other substances colored with yellow dye no. 5, commercial baked goods, ice cream, candies, luncheon meats, and so on. But no one has been able to prove that Feingold's hypothesis is correct—that removal of these foods from the diet improves hyperkinetic behavior or that the addition of them worsens it—and many have tried.

In testing the Feingold theory, researchers took a group of children who had reportedly improved their behavior while on the Feingold diet. They divided that group in half, with a control group and a test group. Both were fed similar diets, but the test group's diet contained salicylates, artificial colors, and preservatives, whereas the control group's did not. After taking the two groups and feeding one of them a salicylate-free and the other a salicylate-containing diet for a given period of time, the diets were reversed: the formerly salicylate-free group then received the salicylate diet. If the Feingold theory were correct, those children whose hyperactivity improved on the salicylate-free diet should have worsened when given salicylates and additives and then improved again when placed on a diet free of them. Neither the subjects of the experiment (the children) nor the observers were aware of which children were receiving which diet. This is called a "double-blind" experiment and is meant to assure that neither subject nor observer will subjectively or unconsciously skew the results.

Feingold's experiment, in which he found 40 to 70 percent of his hyperactive children responding to an additive- and salicylate-free diet was not a double-blind study. Hyperactive children were put on a special diet to see if their behavior would improve—and it did, at least according to the parents and the teachers who were observing the experiment and were well aware of the hoped-for results. There may be some question if they really improved, but even if we assume that they did, was it because of the additive-, salicylate-, and preservative-free diet? Or was it because they had been put on a "special" diet which involved the attention of the entire family, that they had been singled out for the experiment, and that they were now being assured that their unwelcome behavior was caused by what they ate and was not their fault? All of these explanations are plausible. And we do know that some hyperactive children who are not put on medicines or on a diet improve their behavior after receiving special one-to-one attention from a teacher or other professional.

"Well, what *were* the results of the experiments?" my friend asked.

"There was no difference in behavior between the children put on the salicylate-free diet and those put on the salicylate-full diet. Except maybe in children under three years of age, but there were too few of them to make a strong case."

"So you don't recommend the diet."

"I think that special attention and close supervision are more important, and I'm afraid they might get overlooked if all the emphasis is placed on changing the child's diet. I'm not opposed to eliminating some of the additives to the food that our children are forced to eat. But I suspect, based on the evidence, that the effects of additives on health will be found not to relate directly to the prevention of hyperactivity."

The Effects of Iron Deficiency

"There is one nutrient that is lately getting a lot of attention as a cause of behavioral change—and that is iron."

"Kids get iron-deficiency anemia, too?" my friend asked. "I thought that was only found in older people."

"Kids do get iron-deficiency anemia, or just plain iron deficiency that may become apparent before the anemia does. Some very good research in this country suggests that behavior, athletic ability, and growth may be affected by iron deficiency, even before the anemia shows up.

"Research done on animals shows that work performance can be improved significantly by increasing the amount of iron stored in the body. The effect was seen independently of anemia, probably because iron is an important element in the composition of an enzyme crucial to muscle metabolism. There has also been research that suggests an association between iron deficiency and poor attention span, impaired memory, irritability, and general apathy. These studies are more controversial. It is very difficult to sort out the effects that result purely from iron deficiency from the effects of a lower socio-economic environment that is often associated with iron deficiency. However, intervention studies have shown that a group of iron-deficient infants treated with iron improve on basic behavioral tests compared to an untreated group. And the improvement was seen over a five- to seven-day period of therapy, which is too short a period for the environment to have been changed.

"Another rather bizarre effect of iron deficiency is called 'pagophagia,' a word derived from the Greek and meaning 'to eat ice.' Iron-deficient children and adolescents may display an unusually strong desire to eat lots of ice, at least an ordinary trayful each day. The behavior is inexplicable, but it vanishes after the patient's iron deficiency is corrected."

"How can you tell if someone is iron deficient if they don't have anemia?"

"You can do a simple screening test on a drop of blood that measures something called 'free erythrocyte protoporphyrin.' Protoporphyrin is one of the ingredients in the formation of hemoglobin. In fact, in the last step of hemoglobin synthesis, iron combines with protoporphyrin and forms hemoglobin. If there isn't enough iron in circulation, the protoporphyrin will accumulate in the red blood cells—it hasn't anyplace to go—before there is a detectable anemia. This accumulation causes an elevation in free erythrocyte (red blood cell) protoporphyrin that is easily measured."

"Why do kids become iron deficient?"

"Because of the increased requirements for red blood cells during their two growth spurts—in infancy and in early adolescence. Adolescent boys need a lot of iron because of their increasing blood volume and muscle mass. Adolescent girls need it because of their menstrual losses. Also, adolescents are not the most likely people to be eating an iron rich diet."

"Why is that?"

"Iron is found in the greatest amounts and in its most available form in meats, fish, and chicken. Some of the grains and vegetables have iron—wheat, lettuce, spinach, for example—but you have to eat a lot of them to get enough iron each day. In addition, the high-protein foods that have the most iron are also the most expensive foods. Fortunately, you find meats or fish in most of the fast-food shops, but the average afterschool snack is usually higher in carbohydrates than it is in iron. Adolescents are looking for fast energy in their snacks, and proteins just don't fit the bill."

"So you do believe that nutrition alters behavior, after all."

"I never said it did not. I merely said we know far too little to be really sure about many aspects of its relationship to behavior. Food, after all, is what fuels every body function. It affects everything from nerves to muscles. Deficiencies in foods are bound to have an effect on behavior. I just want to make sure everyone understands that a balanced diet of just plain food is all that's necessary to prevent these deficiencies. Nutrients shouldn't be used in megadoses as a medication. Extravagances of this type only unbalance the diet further, the very thing we're trying to get our children to avoid."

CHAPTER 11

The Later Years and Adolescence

THE NUTRITIONAL PROBLEMS discussed in this chapter stem, in part at least, from the nutritional independence of the older child and adolescent. Adolescents today may have their own incomes, and their own transportation, and, to a greater or lesser extent, may be allowed to keep their own hours—all of which give them considerable freedom in choosing their own diet.

These young people are very interested in what food can do for them. Food affects a person's attractiveness: some foods make one fat, other foods make one slim and beautiful. Candy and cake cause acne. Or is it fried food and greasy hamburgers? Food affects athletic ability: a lot of protein—or is it carbohydrate?—will make a player perform better; special foods will help to increase muscle mass. Fortunately, most adolescents do fine. They eat according to their hunger, which is dictated by their growth and their level of activity, the two factors which account for their seemingly bottomless stomachs.

The problems lie in the true excesses—eating habits that impede normal growth or impair health because of their radical unbalancing of the diet.

Dieting for Weight Loss

Until recently it was felt that the only pediatric patient capable of dieting was the adolescent. Purportedly, not until this age could we expect enough motivation to assure success. In point of fact, seven- and eight-year-olds can be motivated to achieve success in dieting. But the heart of the matter is that older children must be highly *self*-motivated if their diet program is to be successful. No one can *impose* a weight-loss diet on today's liberated older child.

For dieting to be a success, there must be a prolonged commitment to good eating habits as a way of life. Failure to recognize that the diet continues even after the weight is lost is the most common cause of failure, failure being defined not as an inability to lose weight but as an inability to maintain a desired weight.

The ideal weight-loss diet has two components: weight reduction and weight maintenance. Most commercial diets emphasize the weight reduction segment because the rewards are more immediately visible. The problem with most weight reduction diets is that they are not designed for maintenance. The austere restrictions of such diets are seen as a one-shot deal, to be tolerated only until the unwanted pounds have disappeared. Disappointment and frustration come with the realization that a return to previous nutritional habits inevitably leads to a reaccumulation of fat. Furthermore, there is disappointment in the realization that simply losing weight has not solved all of one's social and personal problems. Such factors may lead to despondency and compensatory overeating.

"Before you get into the actual diets," said Janet, my now fourteen-year-old friend, "do you think you could go over the basics again? I mean, I know you've said all of this before, but I have a science report to do for school and I thought I'd do it on diets."

"Sure," I said. "The best way to make sure that people stay on a diet is to make sure they understand what it's all about. That means going over the basics. Now, let's see," I stopped for a moment to recall what we had talked about before, when Janet was a bit younger. "The last time we discussed the chain of energy metabolism, it was with regard to athletics and exercise, which serves as a reminder that exercise and dieting should go hand in hand for a successful program of weight reduction and weight maintenance.

"You remember that energy is stored in the body in the form of fats, is available for instant use as carbohydrates (glucose and glycogen), and is not readily available as protein. Protein is really supposed to be used for cell construction and for enzymes in cell reactions, not for energy at all. The point of any diet is to get at the fat compartment without violating the protein stores. After all, you just want to make some withdrawals from the bank's storage vault; you don't want to tear the whole bank down.

"In order to understand the full effects of a diet, consider what happens in a total starvation diet."

"Do people really do that? Starve themselves?" she asked in alarm.

"Some people have been known to do it on their own. If it must be done, it should be done only under medical supervision and in a hospital. Starvation means stopping all intake except water—no proteins, carbohydrates or fats."

"I thought people died if they starved."

"They do if they starve for long enough, but it may take months. It depends a lot on the fat stores they start with. Remember, the person who is dieting to lose weight is presumably starting with ample stores.

"In dieting, the metabolic situation is just like that of the athlete running a marathon, only drawn out a good deal longer.

The glycogen stores in the liver and muscle get used up first as the body continues to provide glucose, which is produced when glycogen is broken down, for the brain and other cells. The brain metabolizes only glucose in the person eating normally.

"For the person dieting or being starved, this phase comes as a mixed blessing. Glycogen is stored with water. As glycogen is used up, the water is lost as well, resulting in a sudden rapid weight loss over the first two or three days of the diet. The person dieting gets excited calculating how long (or short) the diet will be, based on the rate of weight lost in the first few days. Unfortunately, after the glycogen stores are used up, and this takes about three days, the rate of loss slows considerably, since fats are now being metabolized for energy and don't come stored with water."

"So what does the brain use then?" she asked. "You said it only metabolized glycogen or glucose. Once all of that is gone, what happens?"

"Excellent question. One of the great survival tricks of evolution is that the brain is able to convert to another source of energy after three days or so of starvation. The new source is called 'ketones.' Ketones are produced when fats are metabolized."

"What's been happening to the proteins during this time?"

"Protein and another by-product of fat metabolism called 'glycerol' go into the production of glucose. The process has a long name that can be understood readily by breaking it down into its components. It's called 'gluconeogenesis.' 'Gluco-' for glucose, 'neo-' for new, 'genesis' for creation. The creation of new glucose."

"Neat," she said.

"Well, it is and it isn't. After all, you don't want protein to be used for energy if you can help it."

"How can you avoid it?"

"We'll go into that in a minute. Review: in the absence of food, glycogen is broken down and used up in about three days, depending on the demand. Fats are metabolized to glycerol and, through a series of steps, to the ketones. The ketones all have names, one of which, 'acetone,' is probably familiar to you by name and smell."

"Sure. We use it in our school laboratory to dry glass containers. I'd recognize its smell anywhere."

"Well, it may be of some interest to you to know that you can smell it on the breath of people who are starved or who are on very low-carbohydrate diets. Some of the ketones get used for energy in the brain, some in muscles and in other cells. But more are produced than can be used up. Some are blown away with each breath and the rest are excreted in the urine.

"This last part is very important, because the ketones that are put out in the urine take a mandatory amount of water with them. The amount of urine produced is increased as a consequence, and the individual could rapidly become dehydrated if sufficient water is not taken in. Ketones not only take water with them when they are excreted in the urine, they also take potassium and some sodium as well. This is a very dangerous complication, since the body cannot function for long without potassium or sodium. The heart muscles start malfunctioning because of a decrease in potassium. Because the person is starving, foods, like bananas and tomatoes, for example, which have a lot of potassium aren't available to the body. After a variable period of time, everything starts going wrong unless potassium is provided from another source."

"And the only way you can stop ketones from being produced," said Janet, "is by stopping the breakdown of fats, which is just what you don't want to do on a diet."

"Right. But as long as you know what is happening you can make adjustments. The point is that starvation or diets that approach starvation are dangerous if you don't know what you're doing. One good thing about these diets, however, comes from a side effect of the ketones: in great enough concentration they depress the appetite. This is the reason people can stay on the diets for months. Meanwhile, although protein is being used up, which means . . ."

"Which means that you stop growing and feel weak, I'll bet," Janet said.

"Precisely. And that's particularly bad for young people who are in their adolescent growth spurt. But that's enough review. Let's move on to our first diet. It is one hardly different from starving, but designed to save protein from being used as an energy source. It's aptly called the 'protein-sparing diet.' "

"My friend Louise was on that! It was awful. All she did was slurp down some dis*gust*ing pink stuff every lunch. I tasted it—ycch."

"It's a risky diet, and I don't recommend it for any of my patients except in some cases of extreme obesity. The 'dis*gust*-ing pink stuff' she was drinking is made up of protein amino acids. She was probably consuming only 300 to 400 calories a day. That placed her in a severely overdrawn state, one in which glycogen was being used up immediately, fats were being broken down, ketones produced, appetite suppressed, but—and here's the point—protein was being spared as an energy source. She was taking more protein than she was using up.

"As research has shown since the introduction of this diet, any diet of 300 to 400 calories will accomplish the same end. The calories can even be made up of carbohydrates; they don't have to be amino acids."

"Three hundred to 400 calories," said Janet. "That doesn't sound like much."

"It isn't. The protein-sparing diet is a semi-starvational diet that counts on appetite suppression by the ketones for success. Some people have stayed on it for months. It's not to be undertaken lightly, if at all. Some people have died while on the diet or shortly after they stopped. No one knows for sure why, but it may have been because of potassium problems.

"There are other versions of this diet that are less severe but based on the same principle, the diets in which people eat only steak and salad, for example. The idea here is to eat a diet that is predominantly protein or one that is protein and fats. This is also a ketone-producing diet, since in the absence of any carbohydrates, fats will be targeted for energy production and ketones will be produced. These diets place no limitation on calories, counting once again on ketone-produced appetite suppression to work as a limit on eating. Protein will be spared because protein and a good number of calories are taken in. Various minerals and other elements, including some potassium, will be provided because of the greater choice of foods in this type of diet."

"It sounds perfect," Janet observed, and then looked at the expression on my face. "Okay, what's wrong with it?"

"Theoretically, it's not a bad diet," I said, "as long as there is some supervision. It may be slow in producing results, since more calories are taken in than in a starvation or semi-starvation diet, but I see that possibility as making it safer. Ketones producing a lot of urine must be compensated for by increased intake of water, and frequently along the way a test of the body's potassium and sodium—including an estimate of how much of each is being consumed—should be done. As a diet, it's safer than the protein-sparing sort because the imbalance it creates is not as severe. But it has the same problem as the other diet—you can't stay on it forever. Let's face it, Janet, I could put someone on any diet, and if they followed it they'd lose weight—even if it was bagels and cream cheese."

"You mean people would get tired of bagels and cream cheese if they ate too much of them?" she said.

"That's right. Any restriction of diet causing a regimen different from the usual freestyle use of food will cause weight loss over time. But that's not the point—or at least it's only part of it.

"What happens after someone has lost 20 or 30 pounds on one of these diets?" I asked her.

She shrugged.

"They go off the diet and revert to their former eating habits, or perhaps they go on a low-calorie version of their former diet. Either way, because the new diet contains carbohydrates which are stored with water, they immediately regain 5 pounds or so. This is called a 'rebound.' They may well get discouraged and say the heck with losing unwanted pounds. Or they may start some kind of crash diet. Neither response is healthy."

"So what *should* they do?" asked Janet.

"For people who are dieting outside a hospital, I think the best plan is a three-stage diet, the stages of which are nearly the same, differing only in degree. A balanced-diet diet: reduce the calorie intake across all energy sources to something around 1,000 calories a day. Do this until there is adequate evidence of weight loss, maybe two-thirds of what the individual hopes to lose. It may take a while, so I try to make sure my dieting patients are prepared to see the results appear slowly. I tell them to weigh themselves only once a week, on the same scale, without clothes on. Then I have them shift gears gradually to the transition diet, which will be around 1,200 to 1,400 calories. They now learn that they can eat more and still lose weight. They hold to this diet until they lose enough to reach their ideal weight—maybe 5 pounds more. Then they go onto the maintenance diet—a balanced 1,500 to 2,000 calories a day.

"I always recommend that an exercise program be used conjointly with the diet and try to make sure the exercise is something they enjoy. Getting the habit and learning the joys of regular exercise should be a prime goal of a proper diet program. The benefits of regular exercise to health and personal well-being are almost incalculable.

Vegetarian and Macrobiotic Diets

"Can't you lose weight on other diets, too?" asked Janet. "I mean like vegetarian diets? Aren't those supposed to be good for you, too?"

"You can lose weight on a vegetarian diet, largely because

the increased bulk and fiber in the food gives a feeling of fullness without a lot of calories. But that's not the point for many of the people who eat vegetarian diets. Some do it for religious reasons—respect for the lives of all living creatures prevents them from eating animal flesh. Some eat a vegetarian dish because it makes them feel better—they don't feel as heavy or as full after a satisfying meal—or because they believe it is healthful. Some just do it to be different, but these people are not likely to stay on it for long.

"Ironically, the vegetarian diet has one quality that is essential to any losing diet—it requires a conscious change in attitude toward food. In some instances, this is accompanied by an entire change in life philosophy."

"But is it healthy?" she asked.

"It certainly can be," I said, "with some direction and an occasional modification."

"But you said a while ago that the best source of protein and iron is meats. If these people don't eat meats, don't they become protein and iron deficient?"

"Protein and iron don't have to be a problem if an effort is made to, once again, . . ."

"I know," she interrupted, "balance the diet."

"That's it. But in this case, balance must be achieved strictly within the vegetable category. As we've already mentioned, you need the appropriate balance of essential amino acids for a good protein diet. Meat, fish, and poultry provide them readily. Vegetarians have to be more creative. Lysine is an essential amino acid, but it's absent from the cereal grain family—wheat and rice. Wheat and rice do, however, have all the other essential amino acids, including methionine. But methionine is absent from vegetables such as dry beans, soy beans, and peas, which, on the other hand, have all the other essential amino acids, including lysine. If you eat the two types together, as with rice and beans, you have a high-quality protein source. Iron is also available in grains and in leafy green vegetables. You just have to eat a lot of them to get enough. The one thing that is often missing from the pure vegetarian diet is sufficient vitamin B_{12}."

"Are there *impure* vegetarian diets?" Janet asked with a smile.

"Poor choice of words. No, not really impure, just not strictly vegetarian. Lactoovovegetarians—now there's a word for you—drink milk (lacto), eat eggs (ovo) and vegetables. They get enough of everything, assuming they balance their protein intake. They get vitamin B_{12} from the milk. There are also vegetarians who won't eat eggs but will drink milk. And, as we said, there are strict vegetarians who will eat nothing of animal origin. They're the ones who need vitamin B_{12} supplementation. They can get it in B_{12} fortified foods or in special fermented soybean foods which have an increased amount of vitamin B_{12}."

"What happens if you don't get enough vitamin B_{12}?"

"You can develop a particular kind of anemia and, through an unknown mechanism, neurologic disease, which causes a loss of reflexes, memory loss, and apathy. Such conditions may take quite a while to show up in someone who has just embarked on a strictly vegetarian diet. Former meat eaters have B_{12} stored up in their bodies. However, if a strict vegetarian mother decides to breast-feed her baby, the B_{12} deficiency will show up much sooner, since the baby doesn't start out with the same well-stocked B_{12} storeroom that we have.

"The strict vegetarian also tends to be low in vitamin B_6 and some of the minerals—calcium, iron, and zinc—if the right mixture of vegetables is not eaten. With some effort, enough calcium can be provided via cooked greens, beans, seeds, and nuts. Iron, as we said, is available in grains and leafy greens. Zinc is found in good supply in whole-grain products and beans. I should mention that iron from vegetable sources is absorbed better when fruits high in vitamin C are also eaten."

"Do you get any fat at all in a vegetarian diet?"

"Sure. Nuts and seeds are high in fat. They also provide iron and B vitamins other than B_{12}. Whole grains, on the other hand, are a good source of carbohydrate and protein. It's all there. But if anyone tells me they are interested in going on a vegetarian diet, I always suggest they read up on it or talk to a nutritionist before starting. I also suggest that after a few months they see a doctor for a blood test, just to make a count of red blood cells and make sure they're not anemic."

"Why do so many parents frown on a vegetarian diet?" Janet asked. "A lot of parents get real upset if their kids go on one."

"Well, for some kids, upsetting their parents may be one, perhaps unconscious, motivation for going on the diet. Some adolescents become vegetarians as an expression of recently found independence—it's their liberation from childhood, so to speak. The point is not lost on their parents, who see it as a rejection of the things they stand for. My advice to such parents is to accept this manifestation of liberation as gracefully as they can and see to it that their son or daughter receives the necessary nutritional advice to make the diet safe. It can, after all, be a healthful regimen—and, even as a symbol of liberation, a lot less worrisome than, say, free-fall parachute jumping."

"That's true enough," Janet laughed. "But let me tell you about my friend Louise. She went on a macrobiotic diet. You know, the one where you start at a minus three level and progress through the various levels of self-purification until you reach a stage of plus seven. It's a kind of Zen Buddhist thing. She started out eating animal products and vegetables, and some fruits, too, I think. But at the end of the diet, she was drinking only a special tea and eating only brown rice. Now that can't be healthy."

"In the upper reaches of that diet, it certainly isn't, once again because the diet is too unbalanced. Eating only rice means that the type of protein you're taking in isn't complete. No fruit means a lack of vitamin C. It also means that you are restricting your caloric intake.

"I don't mean to put down the spiritual aspects of Zen macrobiotics," I continued. "What I know of it, which is admittedly very little, I find appealing. But from a purely nutritional point of view it's a very dangerous diet if carried to the extreme. Nutritionally it would be no different from another diet I heard of recently, one made up entirely of fruit. The person went on it to lose weight, and she did. But because of severe lack of protein in the diet she also lost strength and began to lose hair. She also developed very bad acne, probably from zinc deficiency.

"I'm inclined to agree with those philosophies that consider the body as something of a temple. But as a temple our body should be honored by being well maintained. It should never be nutritionally defiled."

Fast Foods

"One other question," said Janet. "What about fast foods? I mean, you know, when I get a chance to eat with my friends, or just to meet them, I always go where the fast food is. At least there you get a balanced diet," she concluded.

"Oh? Let's look at what you would get if your diet were to consist only of the most popular fast foods: hot dogs, hamburgers, fish fillets, fried chicken. Cereals and/or grains are not much in evidence. Let's face it, the rolls used with most of these hamburgers and hot dogs are made of pretty refined flour. You certainly won't find whole grains at your local fast-food shop. Green vegetables? Only lettuce. Other vegetables? French fries, maybe a pickle slice. Fruits? A tomato slice, maybe. Or fruit pie. The final tally: poor in vegetables, grains, and fruits. So the end result is the potential for deficiencies in vitamin C (from lack of fruits), vitamin A (from lack of dark green leafy vegetables, carrots, sweet potatoes, tomatoes, and corn), and folic acid (also from lack of dark green edible leaves). A fast-food diet is also high in salt and calories."

"Aw, c'mon. It's not as bad as all that," she said. "You make a burger joint sound like a deathtrap."

"Not at all. The so-called fast foods won't kill you. Or even hurt you, if you use common sense. You'd have to eat little else besides fast foods for every meal to really get into trouble. But remember, those meals are high in calories, and they definitely need supplementation with fresh fruits and vegetables. Look at it this way: once in a while is okay, but you couldn't remain healthy on fast foods exclusively."

"But you know," she persisted, "it's sometimes the only kind of meal I can afford away from home."

"No doubt about it. The price is right, at least in comparison with other kinds of restaurants. Fast-food places actually serve a pretty good meal for what it costs," I said. "And for many families, it's just about the only kind of restaurant they can go to together without going bankrupt. But people your age can end up eating there too often. That's when it can get to be a problem—nutritionally speaking, of course."

Anorexia Nervosa

We turn now to a rare but extremely dangerous consequence of dietary imbalance—anorexia nervosa. Although ultimately the result of nutritional imbalance, most experts consider the underlying problem to be psychological.

"What exactly is *anorexia nervosa*?" asked Janet.

"How do you want it defined—by signs and symptoms or by cause?" I asked in turn.

"You don't seem so sure about the cause, so tell me at least what it looks like. Who's affected, for starters?"

"Mainly adolescent girls, although boys are not always spared. It occurs most often between the ages of nine and sixteen, but it also sometimes occurs in adults. It seems to be increasing in frequency, particularly over the past ten years."

"How do you know if you have it?"

"If you know you have it, that in itself is a good sign. It starts when a person who thinks she's too fat goes on a diet. Mind you, she may or may not be fat, but she thinks she is, and she continues to think so even after she's lost 25 to 30 percent of her body weight. Imagine someone who normally weighs 115 pounds losing 30 of them, ending up at 85 pounds, and still thinking she is overweight."

"Can't these people look in a mirror?"

"It doesn't help. They still feel they're fat. And they are particularly afraid that if they eat what you and I would consider a normal diet, they will become even fatter."

"They must look awful!"

"Some of them do. They acquire the features of the pitifully undernourished: bony faces, bony legs, no excessive tissue anywhere. They look like victims of a famine. However, some may look relatively normal, at least in the early stages of the condition. Sometimes patients with this disease who are diagnosed early on are as hard to treat as those diagnosed in the advanced stages. The former find it easier than the latter to delude themselves that they are not sick."

"If they don't look wasted away, how else can you identify them?"

"Sometimes, just by talking with them. If I'm sitting in my office talking to a person who seems to be of normal weight, or maybe even skinny, and that person begins to complain seriously and bitterly about being terribly overweight, and talking about being on this diet, and so on, a warning light goes on in my head. There are other signs, too. Patients with anorexia nervosa go into what can only be described as a hibernating state. It's as if the body were doing everything in its power to save energy, which is appropriate, since almost no energy-producing food is being consumed. They may even develop increased body hair on their backs and extremities. No, it doesn't look like a bear's, but it's not like normal hair, either; it's fine and silky. Their body temperature drops. About 98 degrees Fahrenheit is normal. Anorectics may go as low as 96 degrees Fahrenheit. Their pulse rate slows down, sometimes to as slow as 40, and their extremities become abnormally cool. Their blood pressure becomes very low, to the extent that some patients may go into shock. And, if they are adolescent girls, they stop having their period, or it may not start. In short, their bodies adapt to starvation by trying to preserve energy. If they were able to slow down and sleep, it would help. But instead, they become hyperactive, as if they had excessive energy. They may also become obsessed with exercise as a means to further weight loss. One patient of mine was doing literally hundreds of sit-ups a day."

"Gee. They must just hate food."

"Quite the contrary. They have an aversion to eating food, but they don't hate it. They become obsessed with it. They can't stop talking about it. They can't keep away from it. They plan menus, work in restaurants, help in the kitchen, maybe even throw everyone else out of the kitchen so they can be alone with their obsession. All they think about is food.

"Yet they put themselves on a diet that becomes progressively more restricted. They become extremely upset if anyone tries to interfere with their diet. They emphatically discount the opinion of anyone who says that they are underweight or should eat more. That person's opinion is no longer to be trusted. Most of the time, other family members are targeted as people to be regarded with suspicion. Anorectics become highly secretive about their efforts to stay thin. They may insist upon eating alone to avoid conflict at the dinner table. They begin to sneak away to do their weight-losing exercises so that no one else will be aware that they are doing them."

"So they love food but almost never eat it."

"Most of the time this is so, but not always. Sometimes a patient with anorexia nervosa will stuff herself with food, maybe only for a single day, and then be so overridden with guilt that she will not eat at all for several days running. This is what's called 'bulimia.' Some will gorge themselves and then make themselves vomit."

"I feel so sorry for people like that. It's so terrible and scary. They sound so driven."

"They are, and in our frustration with their refusal to let us help them, we sometimes forget what a horrible psychological conflict is going on inside them. The parents have the hardest time with this."

"What's the story with the parents? Are they a source of the problem?"

"That's a very difficult question to answer. Although anorexia nervosa is commonly considered a psychological problem, some doctors very strongly believe that it is caused by a hormonal imbalance. If that theory is true, the family is certainly not to blame, which is not to say the family's attitude couldn't be a contributing factor once things got going.

"There is a certain inexorable quality to the disease. It's as if there is a point in its progression before which its victims can stop the process if they get the help they need and after which they seem unable to."

"When's that point?"

"I have no idea. It's like swimming in a river and being pulled downstream to a waterfall. At some point along the way, depending on your own strength you could still manage to swim to shore. But there is a point, different for each of us, beyond which the pull of the current is just too strong."

"Do you think it's hormonal?" asked Janet.

"No more than all of our behavior is 'hormonally' influenced. I think it's psychological. Many psychiatrists believe the problem in female adolescents is a failure to adjust to growing up. As a young girl grows up, she sees her body changing in form and function and becoming that of a woman. The change interferes with her closeness to her father, who finds it more and more difficult, because of her changing sexuality, to relate to her as he did when she was a child. He may consequently send out signals of rejection or at least distancing. She may have ambivalent feelings toward him as well, and these feelings may interfere with her interaction with her mother, who she is afraid will reject her, maybe out of jealousy. She tries to compensate for this fear. She becomes increasingly close to her mother, but the closeness takes on a certain childlike character. She regresses and wishes to be like a child. The solution comes, unconsciously of course, by halting the progress into womanhood, and one way that can be done is by starving herself, hoping, again unconsciously, that she will stop growing and remain a child."

"It seems to me," said Janet, "that what she really needs is therapy."

"There is definitely a need for intense psychotherapy in these cases. The pediatrician can prescribe a corrective diet, but unless the patient wants to cooperate, there's little hope of success. The patient must be made to understand and deal with the psychological stress that constitutes the root of the problem.

"The best therapy starts and ends with understanding and patience. It is so easy to get angry at these patients and to forget how strong a cry for help they are sending out. They are depressed, lonely, and very often quite frightened at what they eventually come to consider an uncontrollable situation. They do, in a sense, become children, and, at least in the early stages of therapy, they must be treated with the same patient kindness that one would use in the treatment of any child who is seriously ill."

Excessive Weight Loss in Athletes

"What about boys?" asked Janet. "You did say boys can get anorexia nervosa, too."

"Yes, they can. But it's much more rare. And then there are cases of young males losing so much weight in their efforts to improve their athletic ability that they become indistinguishable from patients with anorexia nervosa. Some experts insist that this is not true anorexia nervosa, although they acknowledge its similarities to that disease. Others are equally adamant that the two are one and the same.

"The first boy I saw with what could be called anorexia nervosa was a long-distance runner. His role model was a national champion 5-foot 8-inch runner who weighed only 112 pounds. He became obsessed with the idea that if he lost weight he would be a better runner. So he started dieting. Now, note the similarities to anorexia nervosa. He had certainly not been overweight to begin with, but he thought he was. He had dieted down to a weight of 98 pounds. He had a very slow heart rate. This puzzled me. The conditioned athlete can be expected to have a low heart rate, but his was down to 40. He also had a low body temperature. The reason he came to see me was that he was feeling weak. As we talked, I could see he was terribly afraid of gaining weight and was obsessed with food, diets, caloric intake, and the like.

"I was fooled at the beginning. He asked me how many calories a day he could consume and not gain weight. I calculated his requirements based on his expected rate of growth and his level of exercise. I handed him this maintenance diet, and he gratefully went on his way. My insurance was that I insisted he come back in one week. This was before he had lost so much weight, but I was concerned about the way he looked. When he returned the next week, it was evident that he had done nothing to comply with the diet. His weight had gone down further. I hadn't expected anorexia nervosa in a male, but this was what it looked like. I hospitalized him and got him involved in psychotherapy. Upon extensive interviewing, it became evident that he had many psychological problems. He was very depressed and had thought about killing himself on more than one occasion.

"Since then, I've seen a few similar cases involving athletes, both male and female, obsessed with losing weight to improve their performance. The problem here may have psychological roots similar to those of the adolescent anorectic who is not an athlete: a desire to maintain a childlike relationship with the parents—in this case by pleasing the parents through excelling in athletics. Or it may be that an obsession with winning drives them to this self-destructive behavior."

"But is this really anorexia?" asked Janet.

"I believe it is," I replied. "But that's not really the point. What is important is that excessive weight loss among athletes should be taken seriously by everyone involved in athletic programs, so that, if necessary, treatment can be instituted as soon as possible—call it anorexia nervosa or anything you want."

"How about kids who go on a crash diet to 'make weight' for certain sports or because they think it will improve their performance in a particular event? They won't get anorexia, will they?"

"No. Not in the short period of time a so-called crash diet takes. But sudden weight loss can be very dangerous, for the athlete or for anyone else.

"The crash diet is no different functionally from the first three days of the carbohydrate sparing/loading diet, only in this case the dieter spares but doesn't load. The end result is a rapid depletion of glycogen stores as he continues to exercise while he diets. Fats are metabolized, but very slowly. And, in the case of the already conditioned athlete, the low fat content of the body to begin with means that protein will be broken down and used for energy as well. This is particularly true if the diet persists more than three days, which most of them do. As the fats are metabolized, ketones are produced, increasing urine output and increasing sodium and potassium loss. Unfortunately, fluids, which increase weight, are also scanted. To make matters worse, the dieter may try exercising in an airtight suit in order to increase weight loss more rapidly through sweating. The biochemical and physiological results of this dangerous practice are muscle breakdown, dehydration, and sodium and potassium depletion. The effect on performance will be weakness, poor endurance, and possibly even heat stroke secondary to the dehydrational state."

"So the poor guy would have been better off staying at his original weight."

"Absolutely," I answered.

"Well," said Janet. "I'm convinced. No crash diets for me. And thanks for explaining things. It makes a difference."

Adolescents and younger children do not set out willfully to damage their bodies. The adolescent who is obese tries a bizarre and potentially dangerous diet because he or she wants to look or feel better. Athletes who go on a crash diet do so out of a desire to improve their performance. The instincts at the root of such misdirected behavior are actually healthy ones. They are instincts directed toward getting the most out of life. They are also a sign of the adolescent's growing awareness that nutrition is somehow related to this goal. Nutritional education can help assure that this growing awareness will be directed toward healthy nutritional habits that will continue throughout their lives.

APPENDIX 1
Growth Charts

Weight by age percentiles for girls aged birth–36 months

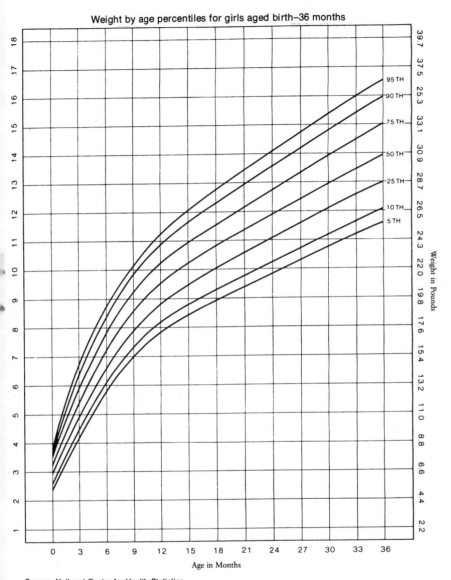

Age in Months

Weight in Pounds

Source: National Center for Health Statistics

Weight by age percentiles for boys aged birth–36 months

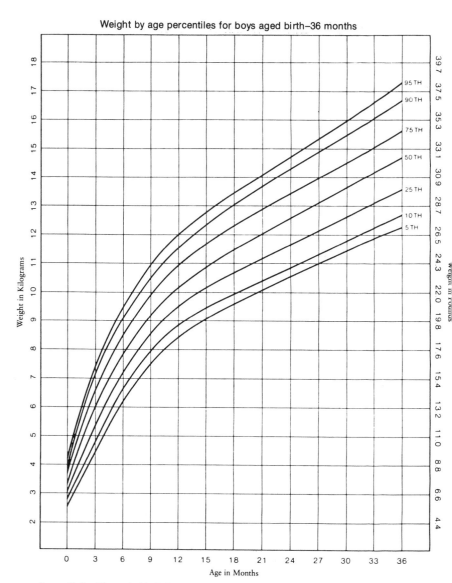

Source: National Center for Health Statistics

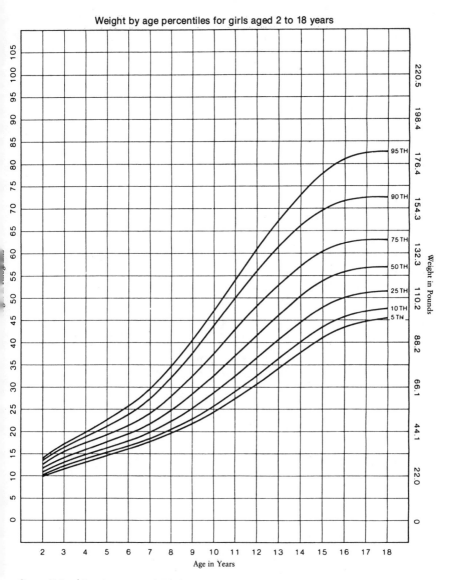

Weight by age percentiles for girls aged 2 to 18 years

95 TH
90 TH
75 TH
50 TH
25 TH
10 TH
5 TH

Weight in Pounds

Age in Years

Source: National Center for Health Statistics

227

Weight by age percentiles for boys aged 2 to 18 years

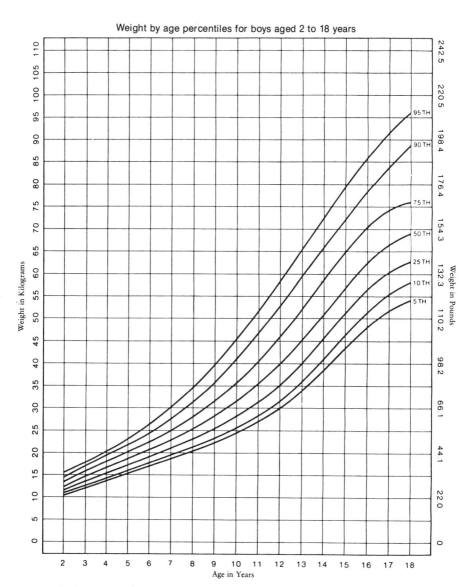

Source: National Center for Health Statistics

Length by age percentiles for girls aged birth–36 months

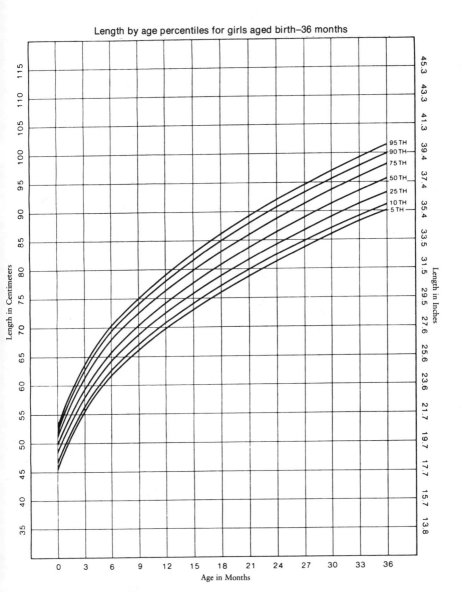

Source: National Center for Health Statistics

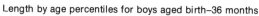

Length by age percentiles for boys aged birth–36 months

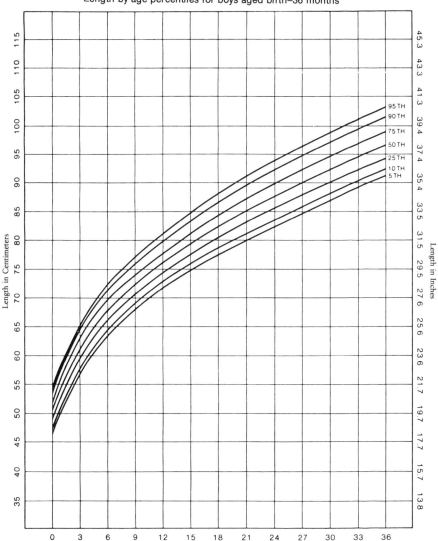

Source: National Center for Health Statistics

Height by age percentiles for girls aged 2 to 18 years

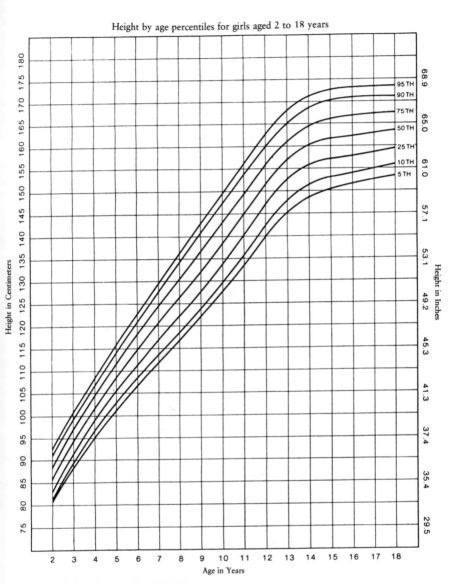

Source: National Center for Health Statistics

Height by age percentiles for boys aged 2 to 18 years

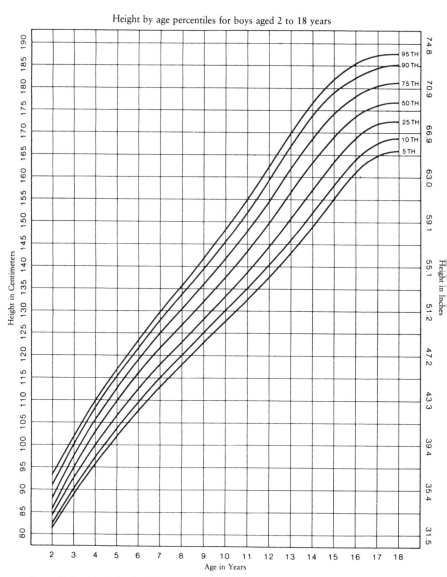

Source: National Center for Health Statistics

Head circumference by age percentiles for girls aged birth–36 months

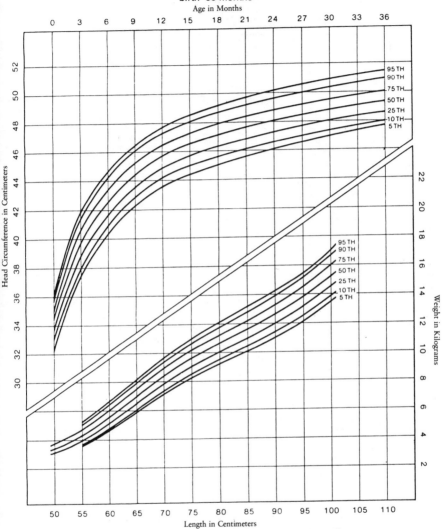

Weight by length percentiles for girls aged birth–36 months

Source: National Center for Health Statistics

233

Head circumference by age percentiles for boys aged birth–36 months

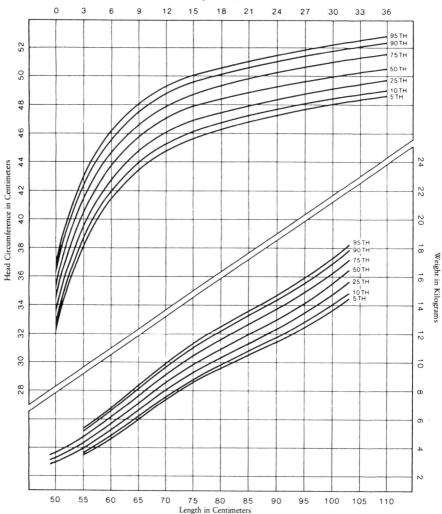

Weight by length percentiles for boys aged birth–36 months

Source: National Center for Health Statistics

APPENDIX 2
Sample Menus

Sample 1,000-Calorie Diet

Percent food as carbohydrate: 50
Percent food as protein: 20
Percent food as fat: 30

BREAKFAST:
8 oz. skim milk
1 cup puffed cereal
½ sliced banana
1 small orange

LUNCH:
sandwich: 2 slices bread
2 oz. chicken
lettuce and tomato
1 teaspoon mayonnaise
1 medium peach

DINNER:
½ cup rice
1½ cups salad
1 cup spinach
2 oz. salmon (broiled)
2 teaspoons salad dressing
1 teaspoon butter/margarine

SNACK:
1 medium plum

Sample 1,500-Calorie Diet

Percent food as carbohydrate: 55
Percent food as protein: 15
Percent food as fat: 30

BREAKFAST:
8 oz. 1% fat milk
1 medium tangerine
1 English muffin
2 teaspoons butter/margarine
1 oz. cheddar cheese

Sample 1,500-Calorie Diet (Continued)

LUNCH: *sandwich: 2 slices bread*
                         lettuce and tomato
                         1 tablespoon mayonnaise
                         2 oz. tuna in water
                1 large pear
                8 oz. apple juice

DINNER: *1 cup spaghetti*
                ½ cup tomato sauce (plain)
                2 oz. ground round (in sauce)
                1 cup string beans
                2" Italian bread or roll
                1½ cups salad
                1 teaspoon butter/margarine
                2 teaspoons salad dressing

Sample 2,000-Calorie Vegetarian Diet

Percent food as carbohydrate: 55
Percent food as protein: 15
Percent food as fat: 30

BREAKFAST: *8 oz. 1% fat milk*
                1 medium banana
                1 English muffin
                1 oz. cheddar cheese
                2 teaspoons butter/margarine

LUNCH: *sandwich: 2 slices bread*
                         2 tablespoons peanut butter
                         lettuce and tomato
                         1 tablespoon apple butter
                1 medium tangerine
                8 oz. apple juice

DINNER: 1 cup broccoli
          ½ cup beans
          1 cup rice
          1½ cups salad
          2 teaspoons salad dressing
          2 teaspoons butter/margarine
          8 oz. 1% fat milk
          ½ cup sprouts

SNACKS: 8 oz. plain yogurt
          1 tablespoon raisins
          1 slice raisin toast
          1 teaspoon butter/margarine

Sample 2,000-Calorie Diet

Percent food as carbohydrate: 55
Percent food as protein: 15
Percent food as fat: 30

BREAKFAST: 8 oz. 1% fat milk
             1 large banana
             1 English muffin
             2 teaspoons butter/margarine
             1 oz. cheddar cheese

LUNCH: sandwich: 2 slices bread
                      lettuce and tomato
                      2 oz. chicken/turkey
                      1 tablespoon mayonnaise
          1 large orange
          8 oz. apple juice

DINNER: 1 medium baked potato
          1 cup broccoli
          3 oz. boiled ham
          1½ cups salad

Sample 2,000-Calorie Diet (Continued)

1 2" dinner roll
1 teaspoon butter/margarine
2 teaspoons salad dressing
8 oz. grapefruit juice

SNACKS: 12 grapes
2 cups popcorn (plain)
1 medium peach
6 oz. low fat milk

Index